True Path to Common People's Breathing, Postures, Relaxation and Concentration

By Surendrhananda

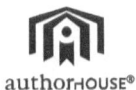

authorHOUSE®

AuthorHouse™
1663 Liberty Drive
Bloomington, IN 47403
www.authorhouse.com
Phone: 1-800-839-8640

First published by AuthorHouse 1/22/2011

ISBN: 978-1-4567-3659-0 (sc)
ISBN: 978-1-4567-3661-3 (dj)
ISBN: 978-1-4567-3660-6 (e)

Library of Congress Control Number: 2011912038

Printed in the United States of America

DEDICATION

Dedicated to all readers and practitioners who follow the spiritual path of this Yoga and Spiritual Book and especially to little Mehir and Ryan and little Mehak..

This book is being dedicated at the Lotus Feet of Guru, the gateway to Divinity, God.
PRACTICE MAKES PERFECT

Finally my most humble pranam at the Lotus Feet of Guru, Shri Sivananda Shri-Paramhansa Satyananda Saraswati, and Shri Venkatessananda.

I am He – He is I
I am within everything and everything is within me. (I-SOUL)

SURENDRHANANDA

Books by the Same Author

1. Yoga for individual Practice.
2. Surya Namaskara "Sun Salutation" for the Children's Life.
3. Mind, thought, Ayurvedic (Plants & Foods) and Yoga for Diseases.
4. Reincarnation, Karma (actions) and Sex and Oneself.
5. Human Body is the real Temple of God.

TRUE PATH TO COMMON PEOPLE'S
BREATHING, POSTURES, RELAXATION AND
CONCENTRATION

"I owe a lot in my spiritual Life
to Swami Venkatesananda
of Divine Life"
WHO FIRST TAUGHT ME
PRANAYAMA WHEN I WAS IN
A CRITICAL BODILY STATE.

TURE PATH TO COMMON PEOPLE'S PRAYANAMA, RELAXATION AND CONCENTRATION

CONTENTS

ACKNOWLEDGEMENTS

I have to thank all those who have helped me heartfully to make this dream of spirituality a reality by surviving in this fake and illusionary world.

My special and grateful thanks go as well to Mr Kalloo and Family and Mr & Mrs M.K. Teeluck for their great assistance, help and supervision in every field work of typing this manuscript in computer as well as the correction which Mr Kalloo has done with all his sincerity. Without his great co-operation, it would not have been possible to realize this book.

I thank hearfully Dr. S. Vaze (Doctor in Ayurvedic and master of Yoga) for helping me also in a part of my Yogic life, health and encouraging me to go ahead with this book.

My thanks go as well to all the Jundoosingh family with whom I have resided for years and without their co-operation, it would not also have been possible to write my spiritual inspirations from Yoga. They are Mica, Nadhira, Robin, Vimla, Manisha, Eshna and Girish and Meena, Newa, Mehir and Mehak and the Ramdharry family who helped me greatly when I was in my long process of illness during my youth.
And my thanks also go to the publisher and printing press as well.

Finally my thanks go to Mr Ahmad Baboo, his wife and family, my English teacher a writer as well of many spiritual texts). He is after all my soul-mate. He has edited and done the complete revision of all my books, without whom it would not have been possible to print, publish and realize my books which are my spiritual message and mission delivered in black and white to all the Universal citizenship.

N.B: *As God does reside in everyone of us, we are all in Him and He is in all of us. Unfortunately most of the modern people haunted by this illusionary world are not able to reveal thus truth within themselves. Without Him not a single leaf can move.*

PRELUDE

This book is being written to supply a clear and methodical guide of the basic techniques of Breathing exercises. (PRANAYAMA) which is the fourth part of Hatha Yoga in the Science of Yoga. It has been planned in a systematical order, which is meant to introduce it among the practitioners in a progressive way, that is step by step approach, practical rather than theoretical or philosophical. This will help most people to practise the most important practices used in preparing themselves for this fourth step, Pranayama. This practice will definitely enhance the quality of their breathing exercises (Pranayama), without forgetting some major postures (Asana), the third step in the daily life of Yoga.

From time to time immemorial, this science of breathing Pranayama has been studied and practised by aspirants, saints and sages who have sought to make their lives more tranquil, peaceful, serene, creative, perfect and self-realizing. Pranayama can definitely bring to anyone, from childhood to old age, whatever the race or religion, the ability to revigorate his health, their relationship and the skill to perform his daily activities. Pranayama, with a little help of meditation and postures, can help people to do something which no other techniques can achieve, after all, it is the only path which can guide people to the centre of consciousness or the higher self; it is all the one Soul, which is in everything and without it nothing exists. The disciples or the seekers become accomplished when they are completely aware of the truth that the soul is the inner dwellers that they are no longer attached to the objects of mind and this material world, which is really an illusion. When this highest goal is attained, the seekers become inspired in the realm of "Soul" which is a blissful state within and which is called 'liberation' (Moksa). By reaching that level, all problems are resolved and the aspirant karma is cancelled or erased and he is free from all material ties and from the circle of birth and death. He gets true liberation. He goes beyond all the levels.

The core of the practices is very simple to study and practise. People will find that the more consistently they practise it, the more deeply will they derive the benefits. At the beginning, one can feel few simple changes, such as more calmness, peace and can face the daily stress with equanimity, However, as one progresses, one will feel deeper and more spiritiual development within one's innerself. This spiritual education is really very pleasant, provided one perseveres and sits and regularly practises it in daily life; this is of utmost importance.

Finally, the practical Science of Breathing (Pranayama) is so pleasant and interesting that people may find themselves attracted and challenged by the other aspects of Yoga.

May thy Lord help you, the seekers, to enjoy the benefits, the fruit of Yoga, that is "Self-realization" in this only human form. It is hard but not impossible by the grace from an enlightened Guru; which is very rare but even by awaking one's inside Guru, definitely one can have this grace in this only world. This is for sure. I have searched profoundly first within, and then the outside one called for me, the Guru to whom I have been always at His Lotus feet.

My blessing upon you!

Peace, Peace,Peace.

INTRODUCITON

<u>YOGA FOR COMMON PEOPLE</u>

After witnessing and seeing and feeling all the sufferings, miseries and stress in human life, I have been forced to do my duty to write about Yoga as a solution, which will help to remedy the serious problems humans are facing throughout the world. My experience and inspirations in spiritual life have inspired and encouraged me to write these 8 steps which are parts of the Science of Yoga:

1. Rhythmic Breathing
2. Pranayama
3. Suryanamaskara
4. Nervousness v/s Relaxation
5. Relaxation
6. Concentration
7. Meditation
8. Food or Diet

These steps will certainly help the material and common people, who do not find enough time, being involved in their daily hard working and tiring hours of their existence. In order to recover all their life force (PRANA), they should practise these above steps of Yoga during their early morning for only of few minutes.

I have come to experience that there is only one remedy to alleviate these sufferings of the common people. They should regularly practise these steps for about 20 to 30 minutes in their daily life as a yogic therapeutic. Each yogic step is a system of self treatment. From the yogic point of view, diseases, disorders and ailments are the causes and effects of faulty ways of living with bad habits, lack of proper knowledge of things, the wrong tune related to individual life and living in the modern era. Thus a multitude of ailments are the consequence of a short-term or extended malfunctioning of the body and mind system This malfunctioning is effected by an imbalanced internal condition due to certain errors in the ways and life style of the individual himself during his daily routine.

According to the Science of Yoga the root cause of an illness lies in the faulty living of the individual; its cure, therefore lies in remedying those wrong ways by the same individual. So it is the individual himself who is responsible in both cases, that is of causing as well as of curing the diseases. But, he keeps on blaming nature, atmosphere, food, the system and others etc.. Psychologically, he looks for a scapegoat; this is called rationalism.

Remember the great Swami Vivekananda says:
"What's the use of building big hospitals. We had to go to the root of the diseases. Then there will be no need to involve huge amount of money in the health department." So here that means the individual should himself find out his own time to devote a few minutes to the practice of the Science of Yoga.

Yoga is not a religion; it teaches self-discipline and a well-balanced life. "It also makes people aware of the foundation for a higher level of self-development and a deeper self-awareness."

As I have mentioned above, Yoga is a Science and a method of discipline that provides man to live a very harmonious, calm and peaceful life and at the same time favouring his spiritual development through the control of both his mind and body complex.

Finally remember that the secret of success lies in self-determination, practice, discipline, perseverance and a proper guidance through one's own life. Everything and all kinds of forces are within us; believe me or not, we have been made from the five fundamental elements which the Universe also is made of, that is: earth, water, air, fire and ether.

And it is up to you to find out the reality and the truth. I leave this upon you to decide your own fate and destiny.

May God the Almighty bless you all.

THOUGHT:

These few lines below will definitely raise and develop one's will-power. "This is also called mysteries." Very often recite them mentally: "WITHIN ME IS THE REAL SELF WITH A POWERFUL WILL. THIS WILL CAN COMMAND MY MIND AND HAS FULL POWER OVER MY MIND. MY WILL IS FULL OF POWER AND ENERGY AND LIFE FORCE (PRANA). IT ENABLES ME TO CONTROL BOTH MY BODY AND MY MIND."

Be alert and vigilant. Don't be lazy and lethargic. The reality is that it is time to awake up. Do it, don't wait for tomorrow; it never comes. Everything is within you. Realize it. Then you will be one with God.

Most of humans don't have time to do Postures, (Asanas), but at least try these Five Yoga steps to divinity and good health.

So with my spiritual inspiration and experience, I am herewith introducing some of the simplest discipline exercises which will be definitely suitable to every individual's life from childhood, adolescence and adulthood.

These yogic therapeutics are for everybody without creed, colour, race and for all ages, either youngsters of old and to both male and female.

There is no fear in these yogic spiritual treatments. One needs practice, perseverance, discipline, timing and regularity in one's everyday life for a better health, fitness and living.

Start now, for God is omnipresent. Perform good actions and then the return will be definitely good and the world will be safe and a terrestrial Paradise to live in. Live in the world as simple as you can, but don't let the world live in you. And believe me if one's mind is at peace and harmony, one can live easily even in the most hectic place such as in the middle of the crowd and most congested place as a market place. Still one's mind will remain untouched by these material things such as pleasure, desire, envy, lust, jealousy, hatred, violence and etc, etc..

Yoga helps to control the mind and to strengthen the body. When both are in good term and condition, you can realize the SOUL or SELF but if the mind is good and the other is not in good condition, you won't be able to reach your destination. Take for example, the ship and the captain, both should be in good harmony, if not the ship will be wrecked before reaching its destination.

Now, to control the mind. You should look about the behaviour of your mind at a regular time everyday, mainly in the morning and in the evening. Once this becomes a habit and the mind is under control, you can do it at anytime of the day when you are at leisure of the day, even you are at work or whenever you find nothing to do during the day, that is when you are free.

As far as possible, don't let any bad or unnecessary thoughts overrule your mind. Always bring good thoughts in with the help of Japa, any name of

God or mantra. Repeat the mantra at the same time with the form of the God. Remember it is very bad to repeat something and think about something else. This is what you may call duality of mind or double movement or two minds etc..

Be very faithful and bring determination in your practice of mind control; with perseverance, practice, regularity of time and sincerity, then you are moving towards PERFECTION, that is, you will come to know YOURSELF. It is useless of knowing the whole world and materialism and mingle with all sorts of worldly and agitated people and insane people and of things and objects, while you don't know your own reality, your innerself and inner world. You must realize and reveal God within yourself, then you can see God in everything and in everybody, bad or good. There is a logic in this. You must have good within you to show good to others . If you have bad within yourself and try to teach and show good to others, this is impossible and it will never work out. That is what is happening in this modern world; it is a pity. But people must change themselves and find out for themselves such purity of consciousness and their own reality and their faithful behaviour. Each of them must follow the good and divine life of the Sages, Guru, the God-incarnation throughout his own life.

The spiritual path to Mangod or Godman

1. BODY – must be pure. By taking light and pure food. Regularity of food and drink with discipline.

2. MIND – Must always think about good thoughts and control the mind to behave in good direction. Always do Japa or mantra and name of God on the mouth and meanwhile in the mind. Feed this mind with Purity.

3. PRANAYAMA – Control of breathing system, have regularity morning and evening with deep breathing, control which is of fundamental importance to the body, mind and to the organs and system of the human body. Oxygen is very useful to each part of the body and brain. Without it, the brain and body won't function normally and diseases will spread all over the body and brain.

4. ACTION – You must do good actions to your own body, brain, mind, organs and system and do first good service to your ownself, then you can do good and service to others.

5. ART OF LIVING – Either you are rich or poor, you must have simple living and let divinity, purity and sincerity rule within yourself and be an example for posterity. Be in this world and let people see that Godman is walking and living in this material world. Each one must take his own responsibility to act as a Godly man. Then logically there should be change towards the goods for everybody and the world as a whole.

For when one does good, this is real Paradise. When one does bad, this is one's real hell. There is nothing somewhere here or there or in the heaven or in hell. It is all within you and yourself. Don't let yourself being cajoled or seduced by demons or by people of very bad and perfidious character. They themselves do not profess or practise the truth. They have just learnt or read it from books and scriptures. Profess what you practice, realize and control your own mind and lead a life of Godman in this world. If the sages, prophets and God incarnated have done these, why can't you people do the same? You have all got the same body, physionomy and structure such as brain and mind; realize this and control the mind which is of utmost importance. Be in the world but not of this world. You create your own Paradise and hell in this world. God is innocent. Blame yourself, not anybody else or God. This world is a PARADISE. See and experience it, you will find the reason and logic. Find time for it within the 24 hours of your own life. Don't escape from it, if not you will always blame others and finally you become a slave either to yourself or to this material world, which is a dream.

Now take a resolution as from now and make a decision for everybody's welfare and for this world to be a PARADISE.

EVERYTHING is within the hands of every human being. If this world is going towards the worst situation, it is due to the misbehaviour of human character. He is to be blamed, not any other creature. Man is part and parcel of nature and he is responsible for the deterioration of this Natural and beautiful law of nature. He is working completely against this law of nature which has been very fantastic and fortunate. You are all part of it and without using the sense of humour, you are doing all the opposite and then you say that nature is against you. No, you are wrong; it is high time, you human race, to know your reality and see God within yourself. You don't have to leave the world to do that or to be a hermit or go to the forest to acquire this divine power. It is all within you; reveal it through your ownself or seek for a Guru, a Real One to wake you up from your sleep and dream. This world is a dream. Nothing exists because everything keeps on changing within every second. So why attach yourself to it. Go and search for the real Soul, the Atma and turn it into PARAMATMA, or find out the BRAHMA and turn it into PARABRAHMA by only knowing the Pure consciousness within you. I am certain of that if you can control the mind by practising Asanas.

1. Good breathing System.
2. Relaxation .
3. Concentration.
4. Meditation. By meditating you can reach the culmination of Divinity within. It is possible only if you can control the mind etc.. And it is not possible if you attach and become the slave to this fake and material world, which is a dream and not real. Just remove your mind from your head. What happen? No one of the <u>five</u> <u>senses</u> will be able to function. So when the senses are not working, where is the world? So get to realize the logic in this, the world does not exist at all. Why then harp and attach to unreality!

Detach from the dream world and attach yourself to Divinity and simplicity. Then this world is a PARADISE.

One important daily thing is that ninety-nine percent of the diseases and illnesses and accidents in our worldly lives are the consequences of inattention to the laws which govern life and health. Remember Nature

(Prakriti and Man Purusha) are the two faces of one coin. So don't destroy NATURE. for your own personal luxurious benefit and selfish ends, if not humananity has to bear the worst consequences in the near future. Man is his own creation or his own destruction. Be very careful and it is high time to react positively. Live a natural living, not an artificial one. Wake up to your pure consciousness. Be pure and positive. Your body, mind and soul are your own PARADISE. As the world is changing within every second, so look for the path of truth which is within everyone and everlasting.

Now I am giving you the simplest form and practice to meditation. If you follow it properly, you will be surprised to your ownself transformationed for the better and realize how long you have missed the real track of Divinity. You can still live in this world and lead your normal life, but by spending a few minutes, morning and evening, on this practice, you will definitely see the change within and how this world is a Paradise. This practice will really reveal your innerself and your own experience as a Godman in this world.

Technique and Practice:

1. A proper and balanced diet: Follow the Diet chart in my book, if you have one.
2. ASANAS :- Sit comfortably in SUKASANA or a chair straight forward.
3. PRANAYAMA: Breathing system, control the breathing. Rythmic breathing Nadi Shodhana-Bastridah – kapalbathi at Anulom-Vilom.
4. SHAVASANA :- Relaxation of body and mind complex.

5. DHARANA :- Concentration on breathing: in and out or on any object or photo of sages etc.. TRATAKA.

Then finally one can practise or get into the meditation path.

What I am defining and writing here is different from what some others have only read and written without self-practice and realization. But here it is all about my personal experienced, acquired and educed from my Guru throughout my whole life in whatever circumstances, good or bad, illness and miseries.

Here one must have patience, perseverance, discipline and do the practice which is the main importance, not only in theory. Mere reading and following the theory is futile. Practice should be done under whatever circumstances.

Please, if you want to know yourself and see God within you and in everything, you must practise the Science of Yoga. It is difficult to follow all the yoga's shastras, but of one sticks to any part of it, some benefits, spiritually and aesthetically, can be achieved.

My advice is that, with patience, one should try it, through one's life, then the fruit will be definitely sweet. The Science of yoga makes you come to know yourself, your innerself and take you to the path of Truth and you experience the ONE; ineffable and everlasting. One become one to everything. It stops one from the dual mind. One can realize oneself and come to know the quality is annihilated reality and the importance of ONE POINTEDNESS.

Yoga is UNION to one real SELF, that is one can see God within oneself. The Science of Yoga is the only path to Reality and to God and within your inner world. In Yoga there are eight steps:-

1. YAMA = Purity, chastity and morality, non-killing, non stealing, trustfulness, kindness to all living creatures, simplicity, moderation in diet and cleanliness.

Non-killing must be in thought, word and deed; carried on with truthfulness and non-stealing. This must be followed with patience and perseverance until the highest ideal is realized.

2. NIYAMA :- Austerities, forbearance, contentment, faith in the Supreme Being, charity, study and self-surrender to the Divine will. One should be sincere to the spiritual life in every second of one's life.

Health is very fundamental to the attainment of the highest knowledge.

3. ASANA: To have a healthy body and a well-balanced mind, one should choose any (Asana) Yoga posture of body in which one can sit firmly for a long time without feeling pain in the limbs. One

should simply observe that the spinal column is kept perfectly straight while breathing in the sitting posture.

4. PRANAYAMA: In this fourth step, the control of the breath is of the most fundamental importance. For examples, when a baby is coming out of the womb of the mother, if it does not breathe, there is no life for his body. First thing the baby must breathe to survive on this planet.

Here the practice of certain breathing exercises will remove many obstacles like dullness, laziness and bodily weakness and will be helpful in gaining control over the senses, sense organs, and nerve centres as also in quieting the restlessness of the mind. One who practises such breathing exercises regularly will acquire wonderful power over both his mind and body. One who suffers mainly from worry, anxiety, nervousness, or insomnia can feel excellent and positive consequences within a few days of practising proper breathing exercises. The main object of Pranayama is to foster the power of concentration.

5. PRATYAHARA :- Make one's mind introspective. If one can withdraw the mind from external objects and fix it on some inner object and bring it under the control of the will, one shall definitely acquire all that is needed in Pratyahara. It is preparatory to concentration (Dharana). First one must be able to concentrate on any particular object, one must learn to gather up one's scattered mental powers. This is the only way or method to collect the

powers of the mind and of restraining it from going out to external objects, this is Pratyahara.

6. DHARANA OR CONCENTRATION: this is when one's mind is being restrained from taking various forms, holding it into some object, either in the body or outside the body and keeping itself in that Dharana state. By gradual practice, one can control the modification of the mind stuff such as sensations, passions, desires, hatred, jealousy, etc and direct the whole mental energy towards one pointedness, then the process is Dharana, or concentration. The effect of such concentration will vary according to the nature of the object towards which the concentrated mental energy is guided. The best results from it are :-

1. Right discrimination of the object of concentration.
2. A clear and definite understanding of what one wishes to acquire.
3. Self-confidence.
4. Firm discrimination, settle purpose and perseverance.

7. DHYANA – Meditation is a particular technique for calming and resting the mind and gaining a state of consciousness that is completely different from the normal waking state. Eventually, in meditation one is fully aware and alert, but one's mind is not centered on the external world or on the happenings which are taking or occurring around oneself. And one's mind is neither dreaming, sleeping nor fantasying, instead the mind is focused inwardly, clear, relaxed and at peace.

While meditating one does not make any attempt to give the mind a direct proposal or to control the mind. One only observe the mind and let it flow quiet and calm and allow one's mantra to lead one deeper within, exploring and experiencing the deeper levels of one's being.

Meditate does not belong to any religion nor is it a religion. It is a practical and scientific and systematic Yoga method or technique for knowing oneself in every level. It is a pure and simple technique of exploring the innerself, the inward dimensions of one's life and in the end reaching one's own essential nature.

One must do concentration first, then one can undertake meditation, i.e concentration merges into meditation. Meditation is the seventh step in the Hatha Yoga.

Meditation is of two types-

1. SAGUNA with gunas or qualities. This is done on Lord Krishna, Lord Siva Lord Rama or Lord Jesus etc. It is done with form and attributes, the name of Lord is repeated. And it is the method of the Bhaktas.

2. NIRGUNA (without gunas or qualities). This is done on the reality of the SELF. And this is the technique of Vedantins, Meditation on PRANAVA – (Om). Soham (with the breathing system), Sivoham, Aham Brahma Tat Twam Asi etc..

Meditation is a most powerful and nerve tonic for the mental purpose. Latent in one, there are tremendous powers and faculties of which one has really never had any notion. One must arouse these immanent powers and faculties by the practice of Yoga and meditation. After having developed a very strong will-power and control over the senses and mind, plus a regularly practice of meditation, only then can one become a supreme being, a God-man in this material world. According to my own point of view, there is no such thing as miracles or Siddhi. This is only because the ordinary common man is quite ignorant of higher spiritual powers. So one is weak and merged in unconsciousness with darkness. He is unaware of his higher transcendental knowledge of wisdom. Finally he calls some extraordinary event, a miracle. But in reality for a man who knows things in the light of the Science of Yoga, there is no such thing as miracle.

One who practises Yoga should avoid fear, anger, laziness, too much sleep or waking and too much food or fasting. One should always keep the balance and equilibrium in one's life. And if one follows strictly the above rules and perform the practice everyday, shortly the spiritual wisdom will arise from within oneself.

When one is practising the meditation technique, it is not important for one to be linked to any particular culture, religion or philosophy as mentioned before. It is only a Science of Yoga or a tool which can be applied to rise above emotional stress and combat mental tension such as anxiety, fear, worry and malady. But one should spend time quietly in self- analysis and introspection within his precious 24 hours regularly. Actually it is not possible for all busy people to retire to an isolated place of retreat because people have their everyday activities. They have to earn their living and make both ends meet. What I call evolution of the world are the multiplicity of things in this world. People love in a place often crowded, in a society within which they have to function and fulfil all their obligations, but still I will advise them that they have to strive and find time to maintain a mental balance by training their mind rigorously and by devoting a few minutes daily to the practice of meditation.

However, if meditation is carried on from time to time, it will definitely encourage man to face the challenges of the external world instead of running away from them; it is not necessary to follow some mystics who hermits retire as hermits into the solitude of the forest or Himalayas and get immersed in meditation. Man can meditate anywhere in every nook and corner of this world, as long as he has trained and controlled his mind properly. Otherwise, even as hermit, he will fail to practise intense meditation. Remember wherever one goes, one's mind goes with oneself. With a true technique of meditation, one can live in the world and enjoy oneself well without being affected by the risks and stresses of this modern world. Even scientists have proved that one of the main reasons for emotional disturbances and mental tension or stress is the complete ignorance about people's awareness of their Innerself. From the beginning of their lives, they are not trained to discover their inner SELF. As they are growing up, they have consciousness only of their apparent SELF, that is one indulges in material life to boost their ego only. Whose fault is this? It is the responsibility and fault of parents.

Through meditation alone can man discover his real SELF which is the source of fundamental strength. Any man can practise meditation, as it is very benefcial to mental health. And it is a tool that can aid everyone without creed, colour, race and nation all over the world.

One must follow the path of ABHYASA AND VAIRAGYA- detachment and discrimination between the real and unreal mind. To realise God in everything is thus the meaning of continuous meditation. Ordinary people should as from now change their attitude and try to incline themselves towards positiveness to practise meditation. It will be of great benefit to the coming new generation and to a better world of spiritualism.

SPIRITUAL ADVICE

First stage, one must follow YAMA and NIYAMA, as described above.

Second stage, one should practise ASANA, PRAYANAMA. These also have been explained above.

Third stage is PRATYAHARA, DHARAND AND DHYANA

THY SHOULD KNOW THY INNER WORLD AND INNER SELF:

There, the last and fourth stage is SAMADHI. But for ordinary and common people who have their daily activities in the material world, they can practise meditation, which is already explained above. This meditation will definitely relieve them of their anxiety, stress and burden of the daily activities. But they must do meditation as part and parcel of their daily life.

Finally, the last high stage of SAMADHI is also possible but it depends on the character of each individual. One can still go and attain this stage even in this modern and hectic world. As mentioned, one must have sincerity, patience, discipline, Sadhana and Perseverance in Science of yoga, this is POSSIBLE

8. SAMADHI SUPERCONSCIOUS.

Samadhi is the state of Superconsciousness. Meditation is the only pillar and direct path to Samadhi. In Samadhi, one reaches the state of super sensual knowledge and super-sensual bliss. At this stage, the practitioner attains the highest vision, that is of Lord, the Almighty. He is fully in enjoyment with the Divinity. He has been the Light of lights at this moment.

When all limitations have been dropped, the person in Samadhi has his soul joined to the supreme Soul. This state is ineffable. It is only the knower and the known that knows this kind of bliss. The practitioner has neither wants nor desires here. All attachments such as doubts, delusions, sorrows, tribulations, fears, differences, distinctions and dualities have vanished forever. He reaches the only goal of life. He reaches God, one with Him, the Almighty.

Samadhi is the eighth step of ASTANGA YOGA.

1. By regular practice of ASANAS and PRANAYAMA, impurities of the Body and mind are destroyed.

2. By the practice of DHARANA or concentration, the mind is clean and clear. Finally by the practice of Pratyahara and Dhyana, the impurities of attachment are vanished and by Samadhi, everything that hides the SOUL is wiped out. He becomes ONE with Him. As JESUS said I and My FATHER are ONE. Even in SAMADHI there are four stages.

1. SAVIKALPA SAMADHI. This cannot give full satisfaction, full freedom, full Bliss and knowledge.
2. NIRVIKALPA SAMADHI. This gives at least full satisfaction, full freedom, full bliss and full knowledge.
3. JADA SAMADHI. There is no awareness in this 3rd Stage. It is more or less like deep sleep. This is like having SIDDHI, all desires are wiped out. It cannot give liberation.
4. CHAITANYA SAMADHI. In this one, the practitioner has perfect awareness with intuitional knowledge and reaches ONENESS.

A real Master, who has reached this goal of oneness and is always in SAMADHI throughout 24 hours, will never make a show of this attainment. He will not even relate to others that he is enjoying this bliss of SAMADHI.

While he is in absolute freedom, the highest goal has been reached. All the past and future are now harmonized into the "PRESENT" for HIM, to the spiritual MASTER, everything is NOW AND HERE.

Even this is rarely possible, but only a very few can attain this infinite stage. So BLESSING UPON you All. Here I am trying to use my experience and inspiration to bring people of ordinary and common background to act at least to the seventh stage of MEDITATION, which, as I have explained above, will definitely relieve such people of all mental stress, illness and disturbances in their daily routine.

There is no need to follow my advice thoroughly, but at least use them as guidelines and make your own way of living and take your fate in your own hand.

PARADISE AND HELL ARE ALL WITHIN YOU. You are your own creator and you can create your own world of hell or Paradise. You can become your own master in this material world and reach Him.

You just have to follow and believe in the spiritual practice and have your own experience. We are all here now. So do what you wish and think everything for the now, the present. The past is well gone, don't harp on it and the future is unknown. So don't fix your mind on it.

Live and do what you want to do now. Only "now" exists. The stage is here, play your own role as an actor and leave this stage. The stage as well will not be here one day, as everything keeps on changing in every 1/1000 of a second. Life is in a state of flux. Only one thing remains, this is God who is in everything, animate and inanimate and He is INFINITY.

Who has seen God in this finite material world? In Hinduism, He is called ISWAR, in Islam He is called ALLAH and in Christianism, He is (Dieu le Père) God, till now no one has been able to define Him, but still people of all religions believe in Him in many different names. So in whatever name He is being called, He is the INFINITE, so to find Him, one has to go into the infinite or beyond it. ONE will be able to find Him, the Reality, with severe and sincere spiritual practice (Sadhana) in one's whole life.

There is only one path which really exists to go to the infinite or beyond, this is the only Science of Yoga. From this only path, the ordinary or common man can get out from this finite material world to the Infinite. By practising this path of Yoga, one definitely becomes a Yogi and once one has become a Yogi, the goal is to attain the INFINITE, in other words the Absolute.

Actually, it is very very hard to live in this busy material world and try to attain this highest point, but by all the spiritual practices I have undergone and performed with love, sincerity and regularity, I can say that it is never impossible to reach the above mentioned.

However, if you ask me that through religion, one can religiously reach God, the answer is 'No,' because religion is not all with the path as with most people, this is done theoretically, rhythmically and dogmatically, with not at all, the interior quest. Most religions have become institutions like a rut and to fear God, who punishes or gives boons to those human beings who pray only by folding hands or ask God for something for their daily life. How can He give you? He has created the bad and good and it is up to human beings to choose what is good or bad in their daily life.

I am not against any religion, but one must try hard to turn one's life into the truly spiritual path and perform this in daily life, then can one become a religious man of Man-god or God-man.

In my books, I have advocated the precious pearl of the Science of Yoga path and clarify it with many practical methods, such as detachment, discrimination, control of mind and diet (food) and have a disciplined life in this finite material world itself. But remember the main importance is that all must awake his interior Guru, then one is sure that one outside guru (Master) is awaiting for him to guide him in this spiritual path and to reach the final goal, the Godhood. A Guru is a must; remember without a Guru, no one can get knowledge of wisdom, one cannot reach God, the infinite and without God no one can know oneself. I mean no one will be able to know the innerself, where God resides. If one reaches this highest level, then one can know God, the Absolute and can see God everywhere and in whatever situation or circumstance. Here, to 'see' God is not with the sense of sight; it is beyond the discursive mind, "above the known and beyond the unknown."

One might be born with a very, supposing brilliant knowledge of wisdom, for example born with the spiritual power and propagate that there is no use of religion or sects, authority or community, creed colour or caste, I can admit his spiritual verdict but if he is against the path of the Science of Yoga and a Guru, I will definitely be against his idea, because not all human beings can have that blessing to be born with a golden spoon in their mouth. To my life inspiration and spiritual experiences, this spiritual path of Science of Yoga and Guru as a guide is necessary for the common and ordinary human being to come out of this finite material world, where human beings are being entangled in the finite material trap of women, wine, wealth, enemies, pleasures, desires, envy, lust, jealousy, hatred, egohood and with a restless mind, trying to satisfy their senses, the greatest enemies to human body and mind complex. I agree with Krishnamurthi about all he has mentioned and written in all his books but I am against him on one point when he said that no guru is needed. How one can be illuminated in this world without a spiritual guidance (master)? Next, how can one study or learn in a school, college or university without a teached or a lecturer. Is it possible to do this without a teacher or lecturer? This is impossible to my knowledge. We must follow the spiritual path of Yoga under the guidance of a genuine Master to attain the image of God.

However, Krishnamurthi, endowed as he was, could have been born out of his past KARMA and maybe, he was a sort of saint in his past life and then he had the chance to come in the spiritually elevated human being with his fantastic mind of spirituality. But this is to remind you that not all human beings might have got that chance to be born here only; one or two larger-than-life characters can have this lucky and fortunate spiritual opportunity to be born on this earth.

But to be liberated from this actual human birth, out of these chaotic and drastic situations of this fake material world, man must practise steadfastly the spiritual path and the Science of Yoga under an enlightened Guru to bring him back to his original image of God, as we are all born from Him, God the Almighty Lord. Whatever one calls Him, Iswar, Allah, God (Dieu le Père) ect, He is the Eternal and nameless in the mystical language.

The above mentioned path is the only way to remove Man from this circle of birth and death and to be one with God Himself.

My example is that all of us can have the chance to come out this material world which I compare like a dustbin where we are maggots and from the maggot we can become a fly or butterfly and to be free to fly anywhere. What I mean here is that we all should follow the precious Lotus flower way of life. The lotus comes out from the dirty and muddy water pond, blossoming freely out of this water without carrying any dirt or mud on itself. It becomes the most beautiful and clean flower of the world.

I am not boasting or flattering with my ego, but I am revealing the truth. I wanted to live the very strict life in an ashram. But suddenly my (Master) Guru did not accept this idea and He ordered me to go and live in this finite material world and be among all these human beings in material and worldly difficulties and be brave enough with His blessings and love to face all these hardships of life, but still do the spiritual practices and follow fervently the Science of Yoga path with regular discipline and with pure love, whatever the trials and tribulation of life, in any hardship with good actions in this material world. As he said, this world itself is the Ashram and the body, mind complex is the temple of God. In fact, with sincere practice from the guidance of the Guru, you will cross out the circle of birth and death.

Now, after following fervently the long path of yoga, I have come to reveal that Guru's teachings as guidance for truth and reality in one's daily life. And it is after having practised fervently and followed with sincerity and love His guidance of the path of Yoga that I have come to realise the (truth) (Reality) of myself and Godhood, the Absolute. "He is all and All is Him."

There is no problem that can affect you or which cannot be solved because there is no problem in this world which is greater than your strength and determination, detachment, discrimination, will-power and faith. Everything can be accepted and handled with serenity. There is nothing which can be called a catastrophe. Treat the problems and control them like your servant and never allow them to become your master. All forces and powers of nature and circumstances must bow down before a calm, controlled and serene mind. And one's mind should remain connected to God, the Absolute, so that the solution of the problems can be found and solved much quicker.

A person, who is stabilized in soul consciousness and God consciousness considers all worldly things and objects of pleasure like garbage. To him there is no difference between gold and stone.

CHAPTER 1

SECRET OF YOGA

"Remember that all religions are good and must be followed with Love. And the ultimate purpose is the same. Maintain same respect for all religions, Gurus and God. At the highest spiritual, all Saints and Gurus become equal. There is no difference."

"To be fanatic of a particular religion or faith is like bringing a barrier over one's mind which can't see beyond one's own fault."

"Unless one broadens one's mind in this respected field, one cannot hope to reach the ultimate goal, which is God."

It viewed from the spiritual angle, the world is a paradise. It has always been so in the past and it will always be the same in the future. Actually, this peak time of the Iron Age, what is really wrong is that 99.999% of the human's mind is very sick, fragmented and people's characters and behaviours are being devoured by animalism or devilish tendencies such as the ego, the main one, selfishness, jealousy, lust, pride, arrogance, ignorance, hypocrisy, envy, evil desires, pleasures, mainly the wrong ones, vice, hatred, etc, etc. If people don't change their way of living, starting from now, they will leave behind them a world such as Sodom and Gomorre referred to in the Bible, and what is more dangerous is that this world will have a new generation who will be living as if in a furnace, which we can call a terrestrial hell.

1

It is crystal clear to see that human beings have become the total slave of their base and unruly senses, as the urges of these senses have become very strong. No effort or goodwill is made to control these senses. So people must practise Yoga to acquire a strong mind, to curb down these senses, otherwise the poor body, which is interrelated to mind and senses will have to pay for the consequences. That's why there are lots of various killings, diseases in this modern world. However, if one becomes a master of one's mind and senses, one becomes a Yogi and will have a healthy body and a peaceful mind.

MIND

1. One must detach and control the mind, then the senses also will be under control. One must have the will-power and faith in oneself.

2. **PRANA**

Without Prana, which is the life force of everything, that is, animate or inanimate in this universe, nothing exists. So one must do PRANAYAMA, breathing exercises to keep the tranquillity and balance of the mind. And if the mind is pure and at peace, the body also will remain healthy and without any sickness.

3. FOOD

There are three classes as follows:-

     (1) SATHWIC – pure food

     (2) RAJASIC – medium quality food.

     (3) TAMASIC – Inferior food

Actually in this modern world, most human beings use Rajasic and Tamasic food. In fact, there are no special dietary rules for the practice of Yoga, though it is better if one eats natural food which is a balanced diet, full of energy. Contrary to what people's opinion is, Yoga does not say one must become a vegetarian, though in the higher stage, a vegetarian diet is recommended. A practitioner of ASANAS and PRANAYAMAS is advised to fill half his stomach with food, one quarter with water and to leave the remaining quarter empty. One must eat enough to satisfy one's hunger but not too much that one feels heavy and lazy; being a glutton is to invite all sorts of diseases, mainly the evening meal (dinner) must be very light. EAT TO LIVE RATHER THAN LIVE TO EAT, the seers of India have known it long before Molière. The research done by Ayurvedic and Yoga shows that food is a source of vitality; improper intake of food will cause diseases in the body. This is why one should be conscious of the properties of the food one takes daily.

In this modern era, the great struggle and difficulty humans face is to live a better health without diseases. In order to confront such a drawback, scientists, Ayurvedic researchers and Science of Yoga are doing their best to alleviate these horrific diseases and drastic situations which human beings are beset with. Even money and worldly materials cannot buy health. Major precautions, practices and disciplines in each individual are required to improve one's health.

(1) You reap what you sow.
(2) You are what you think.
(3) You are what you breathe.
(4) You are what you eat.

Although human beings are taking all kinds of precautionary measures, they often get and suffer from diseases. This seems to be the intractable reality of life; There is no escape. It is all due to our hectic city's life which has become more congested and unhygienic, the water is getting impure and the air is polluted in most of the industrialised cities, towns and rural areas; all these are due to industrialization, pollution of our modern development. Everybody keeps one's house clean but the surrounding area also should be kept clean so as not to impair one's health. Recently, it has been proved that even social care is lacking due to people's ignorance and neglect.

Nowadays, people have got all materials necessary to live luxuriously, but still they are searching for good health. Why? It is clear because they are intelligent in every field, in science, medicine, engineering, the much-vaunted information technology etc... but when it comes to know THYSELF they are still ZERO. Their OWN SELF, which is hidden in themselves, should have to be realized through the Science of Yoga.

"ONE WHO HAS MASTERED HIS SELF IS A REAL KING IN THIS WORLD"

As an overall review, the average human's level of consciousness is very low. Human has descended into the last degradation. He is a slave to this modern and artificial life and live on fake hopes and illusions. He is living a life of ignorance by experiencing joy and sorrow, success and failure, love and hatred without ever realizing the Highest Realisation.

The greatest aberration is that the whole of mankind is led, controlled and dominated by their demoniac senses. By yielding to noxious sensations and passions, humans indulge in frivolous living which eventually they have to repent or regret. In fact, they are making errors consciously while looking for peace, happiness and self-achievement through envy, desire, pride, greed, jealously and lust. Actually in this era, it is indeed, an aid

5

to ordinary man to know about material things to accomplish material ends, but this alone cannot teach man the true aim of existence. In the world of today, science supplies man with comforts, luxuries, leisure and a smooth material living, but still it has not been able to provide man with peace of mind and inner tranquillity. Man has every thing he needs materially, still he is restless, frustrated, unhappy and miserable.

Now it is high time that man seeks in the depths of (atma) soul or innerself by means of Yoga, and must have to experience hope, faith, will-power and, above all, do spiritual sadhana to have a peaceful mind, knowledge of wisdom and pure character. By practising spiritual sadhana, all the illusions will fall away and the TRUTH will shine in all its glory.

Actually the mind of an average man is obscured by delusion, ignorance, egocentric and selfish passions, but Yoga has all the means to provide man to rend the veil of ignorance and delusion so that man's mind may manifest the divine light of the highest Truth or Realisation.

Finally "Yoga" means the combining of the lower human mind to the highest in such a way as to allow the highest to direct the lower, that is, Union with the Self or Soul – "Self Realisation".

The great scripture BHAGWAT GITA gives a high lesson on the various types of Yoga as follows:

Chapters 1 to 6 – Karma Yoga – Duty
Chapters 7 to 12 – Bhakti Yoga – Devotion
Chapters 13 to 18 – Gyaan Yoga – Sadhana (Spiritual Discipline)

All three parts lead to SAT-CHIT-ANANDA

"ON WHO CONTROLS HIS MIND, INTELLECT, EGO AND SENSES, BEING ASSIMILATED IN THE SPIRIT WITH HIMSELF, REACHES THE FULFILMENT OF INTERNAL BLISS WHICH IS BEYOND THE PALE SENSES AND REASONING", Krishna – Gita.

"Yoga is not for those who fast or torture their flesh, who sleep too much or keep awake, who work too much or do not work at all". – Krishna. `The self discipline and serene man's supreme self is constant in cold and heat, pleasure and pain, as also in honour and dishonour" – Gita chapter 6-V7.

"The yogi is steadfast who is satisfied with knowledge and wisdom, who remains unshaken, who has conquered the senses, to whom a clod, a stone and a piece of gold are the same" Gita chapter 6-V8.

"When the mind disciplined by the practice of Yoga attains quietitude and when beholding the self by the self, he is satisfied in the self," Gita chapter 6-V20.

"Yoga is hard to attain, I concede, by a man who cannot control himself but it can be attained by him who has controlled himself and who strives by right means" Gita chapter 6-V36.

"The worldly man is bitten by the spider of lust and greed etc. Unless the spell of non attachment be involved on him, no spiritual practice of his will ever bear fruit."

Yoga helps to keep one's health and mental alertness in good condition. The ancient Rishis and Sages forecast the future and formulated some ASANAS (postures), PRANAYAMA (breathing exercises) etc, to suit all generations. They really fully realised that people will not have enough time to do all the complex ASANAS. Therefore, they gave the simplified ASANAS to suit a common man, a house-holder, a housewife, students, children and even old persons. One must bear in mind that Yoga is the treasure which human has inherited from his ancestors.

To end, there are various paths to attain DIVINITY and they are known as:-

A. Raja Yoga (King of Yoga) deals wholly with the mind and psychic power and may be called the Science of applied Psychology. It removes all mental obstructions and helps to gain a perfectly controlled healthy mind.

B. Hatha Yoga is wholly devoted to the control of functions of the body and to the mastering of the physical forces.

C. Astanga Yoga is divided into eight limbs or paths of Yoga which secures the purity of body, mind and soul and final communion with God. The eight limbs are as follows:-

1. Yama – kindness, truth and non stealing quality.
2. Niyama – purity of body and mind.
3. Asana – postures to give special benefits to the body.
4. Pranayama – breathing exercises.
5. Prathyahara – to withdraw the senses from the wordly ties.
6. Dharana – concentration.
7. Dhyana – meditation.
8. Samadhi – state of the transcendental.

One important thing to remember is that one can't attain Raja Yoga without practicing Astanga Yoga and Hatha Yoga.

D. Japa Yoga – The reciting of any mantra given by the Guru.

E. Karma Yoga – selfless service without return.

F. Bhakti Yoga – extreme devotion to the Lord.

G. Gyana (Gyan) Yoga – Meditation.

So one has to follow any one of these paths with determination to attain God and realize God within.

It is also advisable to practise these four gems of Yoga :-

(i)   Abyassa – steady mind.

(ii)   Vairagya – detachment.

(iii)   Viveka – discriminate.

(iv)   Sadhana – spiritual and inner discipline.

(v)   Swadhya – study of scriptures and lives of the Sages and Avatars. Spiritual texts must be studied at all times and in all places

It is still possible to live in this world in peace and tranquillity. Bhagawan Krishna illumines this in the scene of the battlefield in the Bhagwat Gita. He tells Arjun, His friend and disciple that INACTION goes against the law of karma. He explains :- a man has to develop his higher awareness, not by abandoning his duty, but through his enactment. Each and every action is related to the development of man's consciousness. One has to fall under one of these basic actions because due to one's Karma. These are as follows:-

1. **Right action** – which brings harmony, peace and tranquillity within one's inner nature (self). Man has been

10

created to follow this 'Right Action', then he can be liberated (i.e have Mukthi).

Therefore right action transforms itself into the highest realization.

2. **Wrong action** – which is based on desire, ignorance and the inaptitude or weakness to follow the guidance of one's inner being (self).

3. **Inaction** – which is equal to idleness, postponement and laziness.

"He who in the midst of intense activity, finds himself in calmness and peace, that is the greatest Yogi and Wisest man." .Henceforth, it is now high time to awake because it is never too late to start anew. You may be aware that time is fleeing. So with regular and sincere sadhana, we can realize the Self within and go back to the originality (GOD) as we are all from Him. This precious birth has been given to us to realize the Self in order to escape the cycle of Birth and Death.

MAY GOD BLESS YOU ALL!

CHAPTER 2
PRANAYAMA AND DISCIPLINE
(The Science Of Breathing Exercises)

Before I proceed with the Pranayam Topic, just a hint about the daily man's life. A man who drinks water in the morning after waking up, drinks milk after dinner before going to bed and drinks butter milk after lunch, will never have to visit a doctor, because he will always remain in healthy condition. He has also to have a complete and balanced diet. That is the diet should include minerals, salts and vitamins of all types. When practising Pranayama, it will be better if the food does not include eggs, fish and meat as far as possible.

God has created humans as vegetarian and the digestive system is made not to eat eggs, meat or fish, dead corpse. So man can live on veg which does not involve any crime or violence. Therefore what's the use of killing any creature for man's food.

"IT IS BETTER TO DIE THAN TO LIVE WITH SUCH A CARNIVORE LIFE." The good qualities of a human like pity, sympathy, compassion, Love, respect etc, get defiled and destroyed by consuming the non-veg food and one makes one's stomach like a "grave yard / cemetery."

Good health is the main core of all one's happiness. A diseased body is as a grave yard. Remember that the three main points to reach healthiness are: sleep, diet and celibacy.

1. Sleep: When a person does not get sound sleep, he can become a lunatic. A healthy man needs six hours of sleep during the night. Children and old people need at least eight hours of sleep. A man who goes to bed early and wakes up early is of rich quality. By nature, man must get up before sunrise.

Nearly all animals wake up at dawn. But it is a pity to see the thoughtless human remaining awake the whole night like an owl and lies tossing in bed without enjoying the dawn and becoming sick eventually as man gets the bad habit of getting up late in the morning.

2. Diet : The body grows up and develops with a proper diet and with a healthy food which contains the main minerals, salts and vitamins. Diet has a tremendous effect on body and mind complex. A man who performs good actions, deeds and words, eats as much as required and in accordance with the season and is really in good health. Remember to take fruit and some light liquid which should be consumed in the morning between 8.00 a.m. to 9 a.m., lunch meal should be taken between 11 a.m. to noon and in the evening dinner should be taken as from 6.00 p.m. till 8 p.m.. One morsel should be chewed from 30 to 40 times till the food becomes fine and well mixed with the saliva.

Actually, before consuming food, the name of God must be uttered and to thank Him for the food. Eat the food in a pleasant atmosphere by thinking of God's name always. If the food is dry, try to sip it with a little water.

3. Celibacy: Actually this word 'celibacy' is misunderstood by many. It is not just controlling the senses of the genital organs because remember that sex is a by-product and it is natural in anyone's life. It is meant to divert one's mind from materialistic subjects and to concentrate on spiritualism and social duties. Continence strengthens the senses and mind and diverts to them towards the soul to attain the highest, Brahma.

It is also meant for one not to experience pain and pleasure. Celibacy can be practised by all even the householders as well. Sex does not calm down by experiencing it, rather the lust becomes more vigorous after having experienced it.

In the same way sexual desires increase more and more when one experiences it without control. Finally, it means that nature is advising one to follow the limits. Let one be a part of this respected Law of nature.

Pranayama plays a very important role in any human life and also in any religion. Whenever one is praying, in the morning, noon, and evening, one is definitely doing the practice of some sort of Pranayama. It is, after all, the control of the breathing while reciting any prayer of any religion; one has to inhale and hold the breath and finally release the same. Pranayama is

14

one of the most fundamental spiritual practices. Through the practice of postures (Asana), one can control the physical body and in the most important Pranayama, one can control the subtle, astral body. As there is an intimate relationship between the breath and nerve currents, control of breath brings the control of vital inner currents.

The technical terms used in PRANAYAMA .

1. KUMBHAKA: Keeping the body full of vital air in a steady condition

2. PURAKA: This means inhaling with the intention to fill up the lungs.

3. RECHAKA:- This means exhaling with the intention to purify the lungs. Every living creature is wholly dependent on breathing. It is quite clear that if one stops breathing, then life itself ceases in the body. That is life and breath are definitely interrelated. No air, no life, so here the proof is that Air is life. One can survive for a few days without drinking water, without taking food for a few months etc, etc.. but no one can survive without air in the lung even for a few minutes.

Take for example a child in the mother's womb; the child gets everything from the mother inside the womb, but once it comes out, the new born needs air independently to survive, if not the child dies.

Life is the period between one breath and the next. One who only half breathes, only half lives. Whereas one who breathes correctly with full of oxygen, acquires control of his whole being. Now modern man through fear, fierce competition, hectic way of living, stress and hatred does not allow the respiratory system to work as it should be; one takes quick shallow breath which in a way is in accordance to the fast, superficial modern way of living . Whether you agree to this idea or not, there is nevertheless a great deal of truth in it, that is a fast breathing rate is associated with tension, fear, worry etc.. which tends to lead to bad health, unhappiness and indeed, a shorter life, with a very bad health during this short life. On the other hand, one who breathes slowly is relaxed, calm, and happy, which is conducive to longevity and a healthy living; without such healthy lifestyle, life expectancy becomes shorter.

While practising Pranayama, this helps to remove stagnant air from the lower reaches of the lungs and to destroy the breeding ground of germs and the germs themselves. There are many factors that influence human breathing.

For example, if one takes a cold shower, it is automatic that one must breathe deeply, it is after all a condition response. Unfortunately, most people nowadays rarely have a cold shower, instead they take a hot bath or shower. Nowadays, however most people spend as little time as possible in the open air or go to dense forest where there is plenty of oxygen, but they prefer to hibernate in air-conditioned and heated apartment and office. So it is crystal clear that they lose touch with a natural stimulator of rhythmic breathing. As modern living does not encourage correct breathing, that is the reason today most people have to learn how to breathe properly. They have to introduce or practise what in fact is natural for them. They have to reactivate their narrow reflexes so that their breathing becomes normal and harmonious to life and health. That's why nowadays the practice of Pranayama is of utmost importance to save the new generation from this darkness and to bring them in the light again. Then, there will be no use of building all these expensive hospitals and clinics where colossal amount of money is being thrown for years and years, either you believe it or not. One must try to practise it as practice makes perfect. Pranayama is a science of proper breath control. It means that enough oxygen in the body can remove all impurities from it. If one can control the air in the body, one can control the mind and if one can control the mind, one can control the air. So remember this phrase : "Breaths are seen to be the most active agents during all diseases; all other things are but secondary and subordinate causes." Even modern medical science recognises that many diseases are caused by the unhealthy movement of the air in the human body. Whenever the movement of air is abnormal due to a bad lung or an irregular respiratory system, the colour of the nails turns pale and there is pain in the legs. Many other symptoms are stiffness of the legs as well dryness of the mouth, split of the lips, weakness of the teeth, a fading sense of smell, pain and deafness in the ears, pain in the hips and joints shivering, yawning, depression, stress, worries, difficulty in proper breathing, infertility, body aches, lack of sufficient perspiration, abnormal second desire, emaciation of the body, general disability, muscle stiffness, a feel of cold, itching of the skin, drowsiness and ophthalmic troubles etc, etc..

Pranayama is a practice to control the respiratory system which leads to the control of the mind. Therefore, these two systems are interrelated, then everything will work out healthily and living will be happy and enjoyable. It is quite clear that man's cheerfulness or sadness depends on how his mind reacts to the material world. This reaction in many cases depends upon the state of the mind, and that's why the mind is proved to be the main factor both of man's bondage and freedom. The Pranayama's breathing exercises are not limited only to the training to keep the lungs in a healthy condition, but they have a healthy impact on the complete nervous system also. So by practising Pranayama exercises, many diseases of the nervous system can also be cured.

Health and strength ordinarily depend on the right way of breathing, but in this artificial life of modern world, people hardly ever breathe correctly. So through the technique of Pranayama, man can learn the correct method of breathing. Pranayama exercises fortify the heart and lengthen the life of the practiser. The correct practice of Pranayama also prepares man for the higher yogic practices like relaxation, concentration and meditation.

In this material and sophisticated modern world, there are many hyper-sensitive persons with weak mind and nervous system. This is due to dense populated and industrial area, where life is very hectic and nerve-racking. There is no time to get a little rest; especially the small organ, the brain. So the hyper-sensitive person is greatly confused and has strong likes and dislikes. However, a little more heat or a little more cold, the presence of a person whom he dislikes or a slight unfamiliar smell or this and that disturbs him so much that he seems to be very unhappy and this adversely affects his health, mentally and physically. It is a quite clear evidence that after practising Pranayama for a sufficient length of time and if the practiser closes his eyes and meditates upon a particular fragrance, his nose will actually "smell" that fragrance, so by practicing Pranayama the mind as well can be conditioned against the inevitable foul smell and as well as from the hustle and bustle of the town and city life.

In six months' time of pratising Pranayama, the results are an inner peace and alertness which is reflected in the person's face. This is a proof that man does not breathe enough oxygen to supply the whole metabolic process. As the whole metabolic process of human body depends upon the amount of oxygen inhaled by the respiratory system, the air around him should be fresh and the lung is in a perfect and healthy working order. And secondly the air may be fresh, but if the lung is not functioning properly, the body cannot absorb enough oxygen from the surrounding air. Thirdly, if the circulatory system does not get enough oxygen, the body cells and nucleus would be oxygen starved and would deteriorate. Therefore, if there is a lack of oxygen in the body, the immunitary system will definitely become weak and finally all sorts of germs will rapidly multiply and attack the whole body. Finally if the brain cells do not also receive enough oxygen, the patient would suffer from mental maladies like depression, stress, frustration, anxieties, melancholies and hallucination etc, etc,.. So the life force "PRANA," in human body is nourished by first oxygen through respiratory system, air, food and water. That's why the air must be pure and fresh as possible. Food has to be consumed in a disciplinary way in everyday life.

From the point of view of breathing, man hardly uses one tenth of his potential breathing capacity. That means that the ordinary or common man breathes only one tenth of his lung. Besides, psychologists have discovered that man also uses one tenth of his mental capacity, so this shows, as I have already mentioned, that there is some relation between the intake of oxygen and mental capacity, so by practicing Pranayama, the capacity for the intake of oxygen is increased and definitely the mental capacity also would improve a lot. The mental control of a practiser of Pranayama regularly, therefore becomes easy. A good healthy condition of the nerves is one of the signs of the right practices of Hatha Yoga, which involves some of the practice of Pranayama. These practices aim at cleaning all the nerves in the body and mind.

In this modern era, when more and more diseases are caused by modern civilization and the intake of a lot of unnecessary medicines plague the vitality of human body, Pranayama exercises should be given a fair trial to energize and preserve the mechanism of the body.

Pranayama can eliminate most of the physical and mental problems because its practice makes the life force (Prana) flow equally to and in all parts of the body.

It also stimulates the dormant powers of man, elevates his mind to a higher and brings harmony to the mind and makes the aspirant feel happy and contented.

However, most of the problems and unhappiness besetting human life happen because of his own faults by wrong thoughts, wrong speech, wrong actions and wrong food. These four are looked upon as sins. The practice of Pranayama leads one to right thinking, sweet and soft speech, right actions and taking of good food.

In this material world, there are people who are unsteady and fickle-minded and can't take decision immediately or cannot stick to one pointedness, because of a wavering mind. It seems that it is most difficult for them to make progress in any field of activity. They only build castles in the air. So people with such mental conditions can be transformed and a strong and positive personality can be developed through the practice of Pranayama.

Finally, one who regularly performs Pranayama would never suffer from any disease throughout one's life. One will always have a faithful spirit and an alert look all the time. One needs not sleep during day time, needs no smoking or any stimulant or any drugs or pills. Such as man gets sound sleep the moment he goes to bed at night. Even a sound and deep refreshing sleep for five hours is quite enough to provide him enough rest to his body and mind. Thus, strong and healthy lungs are the most important asset and a guarantee in immunity against diseases. Seasonal and climatic changes have no adverse effect on the health of a regular practitioner of Pranayama. Inertia and indulgence are the bad habit of long hours, yawning, sneezing, coughing, all gradually vanish through the continuous and regular practice of Yogic breathing. Pranayama. "PRANA = breath and Yama = The control of breath."

Apart from yogic breathing, I am including the Pranayama which I personally do practise in my daily life every morning. If anyone of you is determined to practise them, then you will definitely experience positive effects in your daily health.

Practice makes perfect. That is true. One needs a regular practice of 20 to 30 minutes only in the early morning. Try them, then you can see the proof yourself.

Practice, practice, practice. All my blessings to you who want to practise them. Find the truth for yourself as TRUTH IS WITHIN You Reveal it through the Science of Yoga.

CHAPTER 3

MAJOR PRANAYAMA EXERCISES

Pranayama has the power to free the mind from untruthfulness, ignorance and all sorts of painful and unpleasant experiences of the body and mind complex. So when the mind is clean, it becomes easy for a disciple to concentrate on the desired object and it is possible to make further progress in the direction of meditation (Dhyana) and superconsciousness (Samadhi).

By the way, with yogasanas, we remove the distortions and disabilities of the physical body and this conduces to body and mind disciplines as well. Although Pranayama influences the subtle and physical bodies in a better way than Yogasanas, yet this is done in a perceptible way.

If pranayama is done properly and regularly under the supervision of a master with efficiency, the lungs become strong and the blood is purified.

Actually, most people do not breathe deeply enough with the effect that only one fourth of the lungs is brought into action and ¾ of them remain lazy.

In fact, a person who practises Yogic exercises, can reduce his breath down 8 times per minute and practise meditation regularly. He can reduce the breathing number till 4 times in a minute, this make a man, incredibly enough, to live up to for 400 years. Take for example the life of a tortoise, the only animal which breathes 4 times a minute and it lives till 400 to 500 years; this has been proved scientifically.

Even modern medical scientists have given the approval of practising Pranayama for a healthy long life and that several illnesses can get completely eliminated from the human body and mind complex.

Here are a few rules and disciplines which are generally applied by the performers of Pranayama. They are actually not hard, but as in our daily routine, some time disciplinary measures should be snatched and taken.

1. One has to select a clean and peaceful place or room lighting with a lamp with ghee, with good ventilation or near a river.
2. The sheet on which you sit should be with cotton or wool. Sit in Padmasana, Sidhasama or Vajrasana.
3. Respiration must be through nose only, never by mouth, because it prevents harmful objects from infesting the lungs.
4. Pranayama should be performed 3 hours after meal food. In the morning, after finishing daily routine acts like evacuation of bowel and cleansing the mouth.
5. Start Pranayama for five to ten minutes in the beginning.
6. Keep the mind quiet and calm. Remember with time, the disturbed mind can become calm as well.

7. Do them according to your physical and mental attitude if you feel tired during performing, have a rest and do some deep breathing which will take off the fatigue.

8. Pregnant women should always take advice from a master in Pranayama..

9. Celibacy is necessary for prolonged Pranayama and food should be Satwik. Moderation in food and cows milk, ghee, fruit and vegetables, green ones will be ideal food.

10. Never force yourself while practising Kumbaka, ie. Retaining the breath air inside or keeping the air out after exhalation (breathing in is called Paraka and exhaling air is called Rechaka).

11. Pranayama does not mean breathing in or keeping the breathed air in and exhaling it. It is a method to establish control on the complete breathing process while maintaining mental balance and concentration of mind.

12. The Sadhanka should keep the mind calm while practising Pranayama. Mental or mind recitation of sacred hymn is of great help.

13. All the organs should be kept in a normal situation and relaxed condition. Sitting erect keeping the spine and neck straight is of great benefit.

14. The practice should be done slowly with precaution, without any haste but with confidence and prudence and patience.

15. Either you take a bath before performing pranayama or 15 to 20 minutes after the performing.

16. To be proficiency in pranayama, do not go through books or what is done and preached by others with little knowledge. Always look for the guidance of an expert or Master (a genuine Guru) and do them under his guidance or supervision.

Now before moving to Pranayama, I am bringing the 3 Bandhas, which are very important in Pranayama. There are called the "locking". Bear in mind that by the help of posture (Asanas), breathing exercises (Pranayama) and the locking (Bandha), one can prevent the vital energy to go out of the body and consume it inside the body. Pranayama without Bandhas is not complete. "Bandha means to lock."

We have three Bandhas : 1. Jalandha Bandha. 2. Uddiyana Bandha and Moola Bandha and if all the three are peformed together, it is called Maha Bandha.

1. Jalandha Bandha:
1. 1. Sit in yogic postures – Padmasana, Siddhasana, Sukhasana and palms on the knees either in chin or gyan mudra.
2. Lower the neck in front till the chin reach the pit of the neck.
3. Concentrate on the eye-brows and the chest forward. This bandha has effect on the nerves of the neck.

Benefits to be derived:
Voice gets charming and pleasant. And due to the construction of neck, the ida and Pingale and Nadis close themselves pushing or driving the "Prana"

26

life force to sushumna, the seat of kundalini. This bandha has beneficial effect on thyroid and tonsilitis glands etc.. The vishuddhi chakra is a wakened.

2. Uddiyana Bandha

The "Prana" life force is awakened and helped to enter Sushumna Nadi.

1. stand straight, bend a little in front and keep the palms on the thigh or this can be performed by sitting in Padmasana and Siddhasana.
2. Inhale and loosen the muscles of the stomach.
3. Chest upward and push the stomach pit back so that it touches the spine on the hind. Remain in this posture according to your ability after breathing in, rest and repeat start with 3 times and gradually increase the number.

Benefits:

1. This helps to cure the diseases of the stomach and the digestive organs.
2. It also activates the pranas and cleans the chakra "Manipuraka"

Benefits:-

3. Moola Bandha

Be in Padmasana or Siddhasana. Breathe in and retain the air in. Raise the perineum part by doing so, the stomach also will be stretched up. One can stay in longer period in this posture. This bandha can be done with great care and convenience by also exhaling and keeping the air out. This also should be done under the guidance of a yogic teacher or master.

Benefits :-

It helps to awaken Mulhadhara chakra and the educing of the kundalini. It cures constipation, digestion, ameliorates and finally piles are being cured as well. It is very useful to observe celibacy and the semen is lured upward.

4. Maha Bandha

Be in Padmasana and try to do all the 3 bandhaas simultaneously. All the Bandhas can be executed in the position of keeping the breath out Bahya Kumbhaka.

Benefits:-

1. Prana moves upward. The semen is purified and the body gets strong.
2. If this Bandha is practised very often, the three nadis, ida, ingala and Sushumna are influenced.

I started practising Yoga, that is Asanas and Pranayama, at the age of 15 years old when I fell really ill with complication of body and mind. Actually I have written this book out of my own experiences, thirty-three years ago. But I did not have the opportunity to get it published. I learnt them from Guru Vekatasananda of the Divine Life Society. He stressed greatly that I should practise the Pranayama breathing exercises and Asanas. Since then, I have been a follower of those above pastors and breathing exercises.

Now I am revealing all the benefits of these Yoga mysteries which can be derived from these set of Pranayama and Asanas by practising regularly, I mean daily without any failure.

Now I am defining the set of Pranayama. Breathing exercises.

Few hints on Postures
The spinal cord should be straight and one can choose any sitting postures as Siddhasana, Padmasana, Sukkasana or Vajrasana. If sitting on ground is not possible, then a chair with back straight.

It is not advisable to do these pranayama while one is walking, jogging or strolling in the morning or even in evening, as this may cause some harm. And it is clear that people can't do all pranayama exercises daily.

"MAJOR PRAYANAMA"
1. BHASTRIKA - 3 to 5 mins
2. KAPALBHATI - 3 to 5 mins
3. BAHYA - 3 Times, or NAULI - 3 Times
4. ANNULOMA VILOMA – 5 mins
5. BHRAMARI – 5 mins
6. OMKAR japa – 4 to 5 mins, 7 times with thought on the chackras, from bottom to top.
7. SHAVASANA – 5 to 10 mins – / Relaxation
8. TRATAKA.

Extra if time allowed you can add these also.

1. NADI SHODANA
2. SHITALI
3. SITKARI
4. SIMHASANA

From my spiritual point of view, all these Pranayama can be performed as a regular routine mainly in the morning for about 20 to 30 minutes only. The following benefits can be derived by practising these above mentioned pranayama daily, regularly and with love and sincerity.

      a. The doshas, such as Vata, Pitta and kafa can be adjusted properly with abnormalities or then can be removed.

      b. The diseases of digestive organs can get cured.

      c. The diseases of lungs, heart and brain get also cured.

      d. The immunity gets developed and obesity, cholesterol, constipation, diabetes, flatulence, acidity, audit, respiration problem, allergy, migrain, high blood pressure, kidney problems, sexual diseases of males and females can be cured with all the performance of the pranamaya.

      e. Diabetes and heart diseases which are sometimes hereditary can be definitely eradicated.

      f. The looming of hair and their turning prematurely grey or white. Crinkles from face and body get disappeared. The face gets bright and luminous.

g. The process of ageing is delayed; life expectancy, sight and forgetfulness are relieved.

h. Situation like stress and depression are relieved. Mind becomes quiet and peaceful. One develops the real zeal and sense of happiness and enthusiasm.

i. One gets freed from negative mind and harmful mental conditions like anger, greed for money, ignorance, arrogance, hatred, desire, egohood etc, etc are alleviated.

j. The mind gets the habit of positive and constructive thinking and the freedom from negative thought.

k. Finally Energy Charkas are wiped out and helps the practitioner to awaken Kundalini, the third Nadi force and meditation becomes easy to practise. These health benefits are surely reached by the body and mind complex.

Now the method of pranayama is being described and discussed.

1. Bhastrika – Pranayam

Bhastrika prayanama breathing in and out Puraka and Rechaka are done with the same amount of force.

The sitting should be in Sadhasana, Padamsana or Sukhasana etc.
First breathe in through both nostrils forcefully till the lungs are complete and diaphragm is touched.

Then breathe out forcefully, see that the abdominal cavity is not swelled. This pranayama should be practised for 2 to 5 minutes.

Some special points to be considered:
Be careful, those who suffer from high blood pressure or any heart ailments, should not do this Pranayama.

One should only fill the air in the chest area up to diaphragm, so that the chest with the ribs swells up. Whereas in summer, reduce the period of pranayama. If the nose is blocked, do the alternate breathing till both nostrils are opened. There are three speeds in this pranayama; slow, moderate, and fast. Begin with the slow speed, then gradually you will reach the forceful or fast speed. Don't force or go too quick in, don't strain and get fatigued. While doing it, close both eyes and try to think of any divine name. Aum, Ameen, Jesus etc.. etc.. At the time of practising the breathing in, keep on thinking that the cosmic energy which enlivens the whole universe and which is the cause of bliss of mankind, enters the body and mind complex with every inhalation and that you experience that you yourself also become the integral part of that Divine power – Practise with such thinking is most useful.

The benefits derived:
Ailments like cough, cold, allergy, asthma, disease perspiration of all sorts are cured. Lungs become strong and the heart and head also enjoy quantity of life force (Prana). The ailments of thyroid, tonsils and other throat

problems will get alleviated. The three doshas, vata, pitta and kafa are well balanced. Body gets rid of harmful objects and blood gets purified.

The charkas are being revived by the Prana from Muladhara to Sahasrara and the awakening of kundalini also occurs.

2. Kapalbhati Pranayama

It means the light of the forehead in general, that is the forehead gets luminous. Kapalbhati is a bit different from Bhastrika one. It is done with the act of forceful exhalation (Rehaka). The breathing in is to do with normal, but the exhalation (rechaka) has to be done with as much force as is your capacity.

While practising this, the abnormal part, also makes inward and outward movements and much force is applied to the manipuraka, Swadhisthana and Muladhara Chakras (that coccyx, belly and navel parts. The duration should be from 3 to 6 mts daily.

Some special points to be considered:

Think that when exhaling, one is throwing out of the body all the negative and harmful elements with mental aberrations like, anger, greed, envy, self-ego, attachment, stress, hatred etc.. When exhaling the air, when inhaling think that one is taking into one's body positive thinking like love, compassion, detachment, peace etc.. and fill the body and mind complex with them. This attitude makes the body and mind strong and healthy.

In the beginning, one will feel a little back pain and abdomen pain. Soon these will vanish. Don't give up. In summer, make it short of 2 to 5 minutes.

Benefits derived:

The function of heart and lungs improves. Diseases like respiratory problems, asthma, allergic and sinus etc get cured. The face becomes lustrous and attractive. Diseases of kidney problem and prostrate gland are cured. Obesity, diabetics, flatulence, constipation and acidity are eliminated. Blood sugar becomes normal and weights diminished considerably and arteries blockage are also cleared. No negative thoughts arise and depression troubles are cured and finally peace and stability of mind is kept.

Organs in the abdominal cavity, function are more properly. Chakras get cleaned and are filled with cosmic energy. This is the best Pranayama. It also strengthens the digestion and intestines.

3. Bahya Pranayama

While sitting in Padmasana, Siddhasan or Sukhasana, breathe out or expirate as much as possible. Execute mula bandha, Uddiyan Bandha and jalandha and bandha simultaneously keeping the breath out, remain in this position as long as one can. When you desire to breath in, do it slowly by unlocking all bandhas. Do this posture for 3 to 4 times.

Benefits derived:

Fragmental of mind is stopped and digestion is improved. Abdominal ailments are cured. Intelligence is improved and cleanses the whole body, causes semen to rise up and cure all kinds of abnormalities. This is an harmless Pranayama.

This pranayama exerts pressure on the organs of the abdominal cavity by causing mild pain in its weak or diseased parts. This pranayama is very effective for improving the health of these above organs.

4. Anuloma Viloma pranayama 1st Stage

There are four steps in this pranayama:

1. Close the right side nostril with right hand thumb.
2. Inhale slowly through the left nostril till the lungs are filled.
3. Then close the left nostril with the middle and 3rd fingers.
4. Open the right nostril and exhale through it.

In the beginning do it slowly and after with practice try to augment the speed. Remember that (Prana) life force breathed in through left nostril represents energy of the moon, which symbolizes peace, and has a cooling effect.

Nadi Shodhana Pranayama 2nd Stage

1. Close the right side nostril and inhale slowly through the left nostril as deeply as possible.
2. Retain the inhale and according to the capacity.
3. Do mulabandha and jalandha Bandh.

35

4. Keep in this position unlock the Bhandas and breathe out completely but slowly through the rigid side nostril.

5. Retain the breaths out for some time and then inhale slowly through the right nostril.

This posture can be done as long as one can. Benefits nearly the same as Anuloma Viloma.

When after long practice of this pranayama, one can inhale with much force and exhale also forcefully. The can be done for 3 minutes if one feels tired, relax for some time and resume. This can continue from 3 to 10 minutes. This also depending on one's ability. In summer decrease the time, by this pranayama also the kundalini begins to awaken in Maladhara Chakra. A divine name in any religion can be mentally repeated while performing it.

Benefits derived are:
This makes the body healthy, lustrous and strong. Diseases like rheumatisms, gout and diseases of urinary and generative organs are cured. This pranayama is very important to cure cold, sinus etc.. even they are chronic. The three doshas VAT, PITTA AND KAFA assume proper proportions and they regularize themselves.

Blockages in the heart's arteries are removed and the arteries become clean and the flow of blood becomes easy. If this pranayama is done for a period of 3 to 4 months regularly 50% of blockages of the arteries are removed and heart attacks are prevented. Cholesterol also gets dissolved.

Also the practitioner gets the negative thinking replaced by positive approach to life. Increase enthusiasm and spirit in the practitioner and he becomes fearless and feels blissful. Finally by practising this pranayama it has the effect of cleansing the body and mind complex. And almost all diseases get also cured.

5. Bhramari Pranayama

1. Breathe in till the lungs are full of air.
2. Chose both ears with the thumbs and the second fingers on the eyes and the third and fourth on both side of the nose and the last little on the part of the lips.
3. Concentrate the mind on the eye brows (Ajna Chakra). With the mouth close.
4. Breathe deeply and begin slowly exhaling, making the buzzing sound of a bee with mental recitation of a Divine name, like Aum or any religious divine name.
5. Till the exhalation is over and the bee sound stop. One can do according to his ability 5 to 10 times.

Benefits derived are:-

The mind becomes still and calm. The mental tension and agitation, high blood pressure, heart disease etc could get beneficial conditions. And after this, meditation becomes easy to carry on.

While practising this, one should think that the individual consciousness is merged with the divine cosmic consciousness. The mind should be full of the thought that divine bliss is descending on oneself, that deep divine wisdom fills the entire being.

6. **OMKAR Japa** – Divine word muttering repeating of a mantra. Aum or any divine name in any religion. This is the last one to be done after all pranayama. Concentrate the mind on the respiration and meditate on the sacred mantra. Aum (or a divine name form any religion to whom one is pertaining).

With every act of breathing in and out mentally go on repeating the mantra. The speed of respiration should be so slow and subtle that you yourself also may not be aware of its sound. Or one can concentrate on each of the seven charkas starting from mooladhara to sahasrara. Practise slowly so that a stage may be reached when only one act of respiration takes. 30 seconds to one minute. The charkas are Mooladhara Swadhistana, Manipuraka, Anahata, Visudhi, Ajna and Sahasrara.

30 seconds to one minute.

7. SHAVASANA

Savasana means corpse body that is the body and mind complex are totally relaxed.

Technique:-

1st: Lie on the back with arms on the sides; legs stretched out and slightly apart. Close eyes and breath slowly and deeply as in complete Yogic breathing. Beginning with consciously and gradually relaxing each part and muscle of the whole body feet, calves, knees, thighs, abdomen, hips, back hands, fingers, anus, shoulders, neck, head and face.

In this posture one must let oneself go completely relaxed as a cat does. Finally as if one can no longer feel the body.

2nd One should try and forget all external thoughts or objects, so that the brain becomes quiet and empty. Breathing should be completely rhythmical: inhale and exhale taking the same time, remember that the regularity of the breath is absolutely essential to complete relaxation. Once one has settled down into this individual, he should concentrate on absorbing a flow of peace at each flow of each breath. To get mental relaxation one must direct the complete attention on the breathing. When the mind and body complex has reached immobility with treatment correctly, one learns how to find true relaxation and at that point one will feel the rest, peace and plenitude interiorly. The innerself is revealed in this level and meditation becomes very easy to proceed with.

Benefits are:
Remember that a tense body and irregular breathing are caused by bad health. But by relaxing in the posture, one can avoid all mental stress and

the heart and nervous system are calm down, and the circulation of blood becomes normal.

After 5 minutes of shavasana, relaxed the whole organism is charged with (PRANA), the life-force which renews energy and regenerative forces. And if it is done for 15 minutes, it eliminates the toxin from and cure high blood pressure, insomnia , nerve disorders and types of nervous depression.

8. TRATAKA

TRATAKA – is either a kriya or Hatha Yoga at the same time. It is the best for the eyes or for the concentration. It is a process of fixing a point with complete concentration, till tears come out from the eyes.

There are many techniques to practise it; all of them have good effects on the eyes and mind. One can either fix the flame of a candle or oil lamp. Favourite flowers such as roses etc.. or one can fix on an idol or a picture of any God, Sages, Prophet to which he is devoted.

Techniques:

Sit in Padmasana, Sidhasana or Sukhasana, any posture that is convenient to you. It is preferable to practise in a dark room. Place the object as mentioned above within level of the eyes at a distance of 2 to 3 feet from the face. Sit straight and the body relaxed, fix and concentrate on the object till the burning sensation in the eyes or tears starts coming, close the eyes slowly. The attention and eyes should be fully fixed on the object, only then is the Trataka successful. After a while, one can visualize the object while the eyes remain close. This can be practised for 2 to 5 or ten minutes or one can extend the duration according to his practice. But never force or stretch and strain the eyes; with practice one will gradually get into the habit to see the flame or object while the eyes are shut. This is outer tralaka, but the inner trataka can be practised on the chakras and the colours as well. But the need of a guidance is of utmost importance.

Benefits are:

It corrects weakness and certain defects of the eyes physically. Mentally it increases nervous stability, removes insomnia and relaxes even the trouble mind. It develops concentration as the eyes are the gateway to the mind. When the eyes are fixed, the mind becomes the same still. And the thinking process ceases as concentration increases. Trataka is the powerful method of controlling the tempestuous mind and its thought waves.

These are some extra pranayama, you can add to the first set if you have extra time. They also are very useful when benefits are attained.

1. Shitali Pranayama

1. Sit in a comfortable posture such as Padmasana, Sidhasana or Sukhasana.
2. The palm in gyana or chin mudra and place then on the knees of their respective sides.
3. Bend the tongue to the external ends or fold it so as to form a cylinder shape.

4. Inhale through the tongue filling the lungs with air to the maximum.

5. Retain the air as long as your maximum. Then close the month and exhale through nostrils. This can be done from five to 10 times.

Those who are suffering from colds, cough or tonsil should take precaution not to do it. But advise of the master is necessary.

Benefits derived are:
Throat, spleen and indigestion get cured. This also helps to control thirst and hunger. It also helps to lower the high-blood pressure. It balances the pitta disha (heat) and purifies blood.

2. Sitkari Pranayama

1. Sit in the same posture as Shitali above.

2. Touch the palate behind the teeth with the tongue closely.

3. Close the jaws with their teeth closely keeping the lips open.

4. Breath in through the month in a way that the air passes in through the closed jaws that is doing a hissing sound. Fill the lung to the maximum.

5. Retain the air as long as one can.

6. Then close the mouth and breath out slowly by the nostrils, and unlocking the Bandha.

Repeat the same from 5 to 10 times this posture should be done not too often in winter.

Benefits derived are:

Same benefits as stitali. And ailments pertaining to teeth, pyorrhea and to throat cavity, month, nose tongue etc.. are getting cured. This posture keeps the body cool and even cures sleepiness. And if done for longer time can cure hypertension.

3. Simhasana

Preferable if one can face the sun in the morning. Sit in Vajrasana and spread the knees apart and the toes touch together. The fingers of the hand should be turning backside and keep them straight in between the under the legs and thighs.

Inhale and take out the tongue. Look in between the eyebrows and exhale with a roaring sound of a lion 5 to 10 times.

After doing the posture leave the saliva from the month and highly massage the throat this prevents sore throat.

Benefits derived are:

It is useful for tonsils, thyroid and other throat problems.
It is beneficial for ear problems and for those who can't pronounce clean pronunciation.
It has also beneficial cure on children with tottering lips.

N.B. The best time to practise it is between 4 a.m. to 6 a.m. But it can be practised at any time; the stomach should be empty.

These are the Four extra pranayama

1. NADI SHODANA
2. SHITALI
3. SITKARI
4. SIMHASANA

"FIVE SHEATHS" KOSHAS

According to the medical scientists, Yoga Asanas, breathing exercises, Pranayama therapy are successful because they create balance in the nervous system and endocrine systems which influence directly all the other organs and systems of the body. Therefore, the Science of Yoga reacts both as a preventive therapy and aid curative to the body and mind complex.

The very essence of Yoga Asana and Pranayama is to attain mental peace, improved concentration, a relaxed state of living in harmony and peace with the world. Through the practice of yoga and Asanas and Pranayama, one becomes aware of the interrelationship and interconnectedness between our emotional, mental and physical levels. Little by little, this awareness leads to an understanding of more subtle areas of existence. The highest goal of Yoga Asana and Pranayama is to get it possible to fuse together the gross material Anamaya, physical (Pranamaya), mental Manomaya, intellectual (Vignyanamaga) and spiritual (Anandamaya) levels within the One.

Five sheaths (Koshas)

These above mentioned Five sheaths show that the five-fold body is surrounded by the soul and one above the other, the outer sheaths penetrate the inner ones.

1. Annamaya sheaths (Kosha):- The physical body is that which needs food as constitution and sustenance. This is the first sheath of the body. This sheath (Kosha) composes the physical body, begins from the outmost part the skin and the inner recesses, like bones, flesh, all organs, brains etc.. It is related to the earth element as shown by its denseness. By taking pure food and regular practice in Postures (Asana) and breathing exercise, Pranayama, a clean and healthy body is reached.

2. Pranamaya Kasha

This second sheath is called Pranamaya (Kosha), the other body or Pranic Body. Very few spiritual people recognize its existence. This sheath covers and permeates the physical body of the Annamaya sheath and it is not visible as the above Annamaya (Kosha).

It is now that scientists have started to discover this sheath. It is said to be the possession of knowledge and to direct the functioning of the physical body. The Pranic force which one inhales and exhales is divided into ten types. They are Vyana, Udana, Prana, Samana, and Apana and they are considered to be the principal Pranas. Ref: to my other book on (Prana) life force. The Prana activates the food to get digested properly and to divide the humours in separate elements such as sweat, faeces and other elements and also reject them from human body.

Finally it helps to enjoy the pleasures which are derived from the task of the sense organs and mental processes. So by regular practice of Yoga, Asana and Pranayama, this sheath becomes more energetic and efficient, which in turn energises the first sheath. Annamaya kosha.

3. Manomaya Sheath (Kosha)

Manomaya Sheath (Kosha) is known as mental sheath. It is believed to be the prime body which functions and controls the activation of the first two sheaths, Annamaya kosha and Pranamaya Kosha. Mind, intelligence, ego, conscience, the power of reasoning, feelings, emotions (Chitta) are known to be the essence known wholly as Antahkarana chatushtaya. It also controls the five senses or organs as eyes, nose, tongue and skin which brings man to be aware of the external world and its activities.

4. Vignyanamaya Kosha

This fourth sheath is known as Vignyanamaya Kosha, which contains within itself the elements of intelligence and ego. This sheath is responsible for the sense of doer, enjoyer and so on.

It controls the functioning of the fourth body which gives rise to the feelings of pain, pleasure, love, hatred etc, etc..

One who understands its functioning can modulate his thoughts and actions accordingly, keeping himself away from pain, illusion, worldly temptations, attachment etc.. and remain absorbed in complete high level meditation and achieve the highest state of wisdom known in Yogic knowledge. We can then discriminate from falsehood, illusion, unsteadiness, wavering and other negative attitudes.

5. Anandamaya Sheath

Actually this sheath is called by many names. It location is recognized to be in the heart and it is closely related to the innerself, the inner world. That means that our lives, the existence of the gross body and the relations with the world as such depends on this sheath. When doing meditation the yoga practitioners become free from the chain of physical life and enjoys an eternal blissful attitude.

Now the great yogic sage, Patanjali of whom I am a worshipper, has put forward the eight fold rules or disciplines for those who wish to tread the path of yoga, the Science of Yoga.

They are 1. Yamas, 2. Niyamas, 3. Asanas, 4. Pranayama (breathing exercises) 5.Pratyahara, 6. Dharana, 7. Dhyana and 8. Samadhi.

You can refer to my other book.

First discipline : Yama :-

1. Ahinsa (non-violence, physical as well as mental)

47

1. Asteya (non-stealing)

2. Satya – Truthfulness

3. Brahmacharya (celibacy or continence)

4. Aparigraha (abstinence from avarice, greed, desire to covet things not necessary for our maintenance).

Second discipline: Niyamas:-

1. Shaucha (cleansing the mind and the body from dross and contaminating elements, by practising Asanas and Pranayama which are the fundamental importance for a Sadhaka.

2. Santosha:- (Contentment) satisfaction and acceptation.

3. Tapa: (Observance of religious austerities) final goal of yoga. Samadhi = freedom and liberation). Mental or equipoise, unpleasant or painful situation.

4. Swadhyaya:- constant study on the knowledge of the spiritual subjects. Mantra or gayatri such like Om, Ameen, Amen etc.. and study of religious scriptures.

5. Ishwarapranidhana: (Complete devotion to God with the practice of Yama and Niyama, Asana and pranayama, pratyahara, Dharana, Dhyana and Samadhi.

I have here given just a brief account of the eight-fold path of yoga. In my other book on Yoga I have been more elaborate.

The importance of "PRANA". "Prana" is another word for the vital force, without which the body won't survive for a fraction of a second. It is in the whole body and all cells. Here by practising the technique of Pranayama, this "PRANA" or Life-force or vital force can be controlled and regulated in a way; this allows the disciple to establish unity with the Ultimate Reality, which is highest goal of Nirvana, Moksha or freedom and liberation which is called Samadhi.

Remember that the body is bound by the five elements. They are

1. Akasha (space) ether.
2. Vayu (Air)
3. Agni (Fire)
4. Jala (Water)
5. Prithvi (Earth)

Here Air is supposed to be the most essential element which keeps the body alive. This air when inhaled in the body by the breathing system is called "PRANA," the vital force.

In the Science of Yoga and Ayurvedic, these above five elements compose the three Dosha's humours

1. Vata (air) 2. Pitta (heat) and 3. Kapha (Phlegme).

Take for example the clouds in the sky which are being drifted by the wind force so, it is with the Doshas which are being taken from one place to another by the element, air. Prana has been compared to Brahma, the Supreme Being, from whom this whole universe has emerged. Prana

49

always remains active. It has no rest at all. A constant and active movement is its inner behaviour. As far as the vital force "Prana" remains functioning in the body, the being will remain alive. Life depends on Prana. It is due to Prana that everything in this universe remains alive and their communications and functions continue without interruption without the slightest stop.

No Prana no life; people can survive without food or water for several days but without Prana, life goes. The Pranic energy is a complete and whole essence to our body and mind complex.

N.B.:- Whatever exists in the entire universe, in all the three worlds, within or beyond man's cognition-all is in the contol of "Prana," the life force, the élan vital of Bergson.

Prana is always in MOTION, and is divided into five different names according to their locations and functions in the human body: 1. Prana 2. Apana, 3. Vyana, 4. Udana and 5. Samana, but any way, the Pranic energy is the same.

1. Prana: It is situated in the area between the throat and heart and is known by its generic name "Prana".

Its function: It provides energy to the organs of breathing of speech and esophagus and makes them active. Chrakra is Muladhara and element is Earth.

2. Apana: It is between the navel umbilicus which is considered to be the center and focal point of the organs of body and toes.

Its function is to clean the body of all dross and used elements like excretion, sweat, phlegm, urine, faeces and to render the system clean. Chakra is swadhisthana and element is water.

3. Udana:- It is between the throat and head.

Its function is to energize the organs found in this area. It covers organs such as the eyes, ears, nostrils and the mouth and makes live luster to the face. It makes the pineal and pituitary glands activate the chakra manipuraka the element is fire.

4. Samana: It is in the region between the heart and navel.

Its function is to activate and also control the liver, intestines, spleen, pancreas and the digestive system. The chakra is Anahata and element is vayu (Air).

5. Vyana:- It is found throughout the whole body.

Its function is to control, energize and regulate the body organs and synthesize their functioning. Its also generates all the body muscles, tissues, joints and nadis.

So Pranayama, breathing exercises are aimed to clean the Pranas and Pranayama sheath and make the esthetic body healthy, the chakra, vishudhi and elements is Akasha.

The beginners of Pranayama would have a clue of all the koshas (Sheaths), Prana and eight folds of hatha yoga before they could start practising the Pranayama.

Attached a CHART FOR PRANAYAMA
1. BHASTRIKA – 2mts to 5 mts.
2. KAPALBHATI – 2 mts to 5 mts.
3. BAHYA – 3 Times.
4. NAULI – 3 to 4 times.
5. ANULOMA VILOMA – 2 mt to 5 mts.
6. BHRAMARI – 2 mt to 5 mts.
7. SHITALI – 4 Times.
8. SITKARI – 4 Times.
9. OMKAR Japa – 5 mts – 7 times with thougfht on the CHAKRAS from bottom to top
10. SIMHA – 5 Times.
11. SHAVASANA – 8 to 10 mts/ Relaxation
12. CONCENTRATION as TRATAKA – 2 to 5 mts.

I am here mentioning some cures and benefits which one can derive from practising daily and regularly these above mentioned exercises of breathing.
1. All the abnormalities and problems of the mind and the body can definitely get cured.
2. Mental attitudes get stable and tranquil and a sense of enthusiasm, zeal or contentment are developed. Stress or depression can be relieved.

52

3. One becomes free from negative thinking and the mind is influenced to positive and constructive thinking.
4. The physical and etheric body diseases are cured. And freedom will be attained, from negative and harmful mental situations such as anger, worry, tensions, arrogance, ignorance, lust, vice, envy, attachment and mainly greed for money etc..etc..
5. At this point the Yogic meditation will be easy to carry on.
6. The abnormalities of all 3 doshas "Vata, Pitta and kapha are removed and they get regulated in a proper way.
7. Digestive system gets ameliorated and its ailments also get cured.
8. Resistance and immunity get developed.
9. The problem of hereditary diseases like H.B.P and cardio-vascular diseases and diabetes also are cured. Obesity, cholesterol, constipation, flatulence, acidity, respiratory problems, allergy, migraine, kidney problems, sexual diseases of both sex are definitely cured.
10. Lungs and brain diseases are also cured.
11. Falling of hair and their turning prematurely grey and white, wrinkles on the face or on other part of the body, weak eye-sight, forgetfulness are all alleviated and the ageing in man is being retarded as well.
12. If one has any idea of chakras and kundalini, then one can feel the energy of chakras is cleansed and the kundalini is awakened.
13. Finally the face becomes luminous and bright.

If the practice is done daily and regularly after a few weeks, one can notice the beneficial and tremendous changes of Pranayama and it's mysteries.

CHAPTER 4
YOGIC AND RHYTHMIC BREATHING

WAYS TO HAPPINESS AND HEALTHY LIVING

PRANAYAMA:-

PRANA is a vital force, cosmic energy. Ayana is the control of Prana. Hence, PRANAYAMA is the control of the vital force by regulating the breath with concentration. Actually, two main processes are of fundamental importance to life:

1. The absorption of air by the inhalation of oxygen.
2. The expulsion by the exhalation of carbonic gas.

Even when the body is at rest, it is constantly at work. The organs and body system such as blood circulation, respiratory, endocrine, digestive and nervous systems are all automatically in operation. Nourishment must be fed to repair the losses such as wear and tear of the body. This does not come only from food and drink, but also from the air one breathes. It is crystal clear that oxygen is of a fundamental part of food. Survival is impossible without oxygen, even for a fraction of a few seconds. After all, not only the digestion needs oxygen, but all the system of the body is in need of the oxygen we breathe. "So without Air nothing will move and survive on this Universe". Air is indispensable.

Breath is ever-present and it is clear that when a child is born, if it does not breathe it dies. So breath is life. Remember that life is nothing, but a sequence of breathing. Most people develop respiratory illnesses due to short and wrong way of breathing. It has been investigated by scientists and doctors that unsatisfactory breathing habits diminish the resistance and shorten life.

Vivekananda says:
"From thought down to the lowest force, everything is but only the manifestation of Prana(Life force). The sum total of all forces in the universe, mental or physical, when resolved back to their state is called Prana."

Without it nothing exists, either life or the universe. Even in the Bible, we have: "When the Almighty God created first man, breath was blown first to give life to Adam."

"And Lord God formed man of the dust of the ground and breathed into the nostril the breath of life and man become, all living soul."

From the yogic point of view, a yogi does not measure his life span by the number of years, months, weeks and days, but astonishingly by the number of his breaths.

So a complete yogic breathing contains three parts:
1. Abdominal breathing.
2. Middle part of the chest thorax breathing.

3. Upper part of the chest collar bones, clavicle breathing.

N.B. Inhale and exhale should be done only through the nose.

1. **Abdominal breathing**: One can stand, sit crossed-legged or lying on one's back. The method is to rest the hands softly on the abdomen so that the movement of the breaths may be felt. During inhalation, the abdomen should be allowed to expand a little, like a bow, as the lower part of the lung is filled with air. While exhalation, the abdomen is felt to sink in again. This process should be repeated several times.

2. **Breathing from the thorax middle part of chest.** Lying on the back, sitting or standing. Rest both hands on either side of the ribs cage softly, inhale slowly inflating the sides then contract them by exhaling like an accordeon and repeat several times.

3. **Breathing from the Clavicle (Upper part of chest).** Lying on the back, sitting or standing. Rest the hands on each side of the clavide touching it with the fingers. Contract slightly the stomach. Inhale slowly pushing the clavicle or collar bones upwards, then begin to exhale pushing it downwards. Repeat several times.

2. Complete Yogic breathing standing, lying on back or sitting crossed-legged.

In this complete Yogic breathing, the three parts are combined altogether, that is abdominal, thorax and clavicle parts and this makes a wave-like movement.

After exhaling completely, begin to inhale letting the abdomen come out a little and filling the lower part of the lungs, then expanding the ribs, whilst slightly drawing in the stomach until finally fill the top part of the lungs, that is the collar bones raise upwards.

Now exhalation begins with the abdomen being drawn when the ribs are contracted and finally the collar bone lowered, then completely emptying the lungs.

The complete process of inhaling and exhaling should be done as one smooth, continuous movement, like a wave on the surface of the sea which one might have noticed. And the volume of breath while inhaling should be the same.

It seems quite difficult to breathe with gentle, continuous movement, but once the habit is acquired, this wave-like breathing becomes almost natural. It is only with little practice, patience and perseverance that the beneficial results will be attained.

3. Now the 3rd Rhythmic Breathing. This item is not difficult, so every one can do it. There are two variations in rhythmic breathing:

1. First variation:- Inhale from the complete yogic breathing, mentally counting 4 heartbeats, then slowly exhale through the nostrils again counting 4 heart beats mentally. Repeat several times. Or while walking one can do it as well. Counting 4 steps while inhaling and counting 4 steps while exhaling.

2. Second variation: The posture is the same except one has to inhale and counting from 1 to 6, the breath should be held from 1 to 3, then exhale again 1 to 6 and remain without breathing to a counting of 1 to 3, then start again to inhale etc.. The beginner should concentrate particularly on acquiring a rhythmic breathing pattern without forcing or straining to prolong the duration of inhalation and exhalation. It is only after long practice that one will be able to come up to 10 or 12 or 16 beats instead of 6 beats.

3. The retention of the breath. (Kumbhakas) sitting cross-legged or in the lotus posture, inhale as in complete yogic breathing, then holds the breath from six to thirty two seconds, adding one second each day, till the maximum of thirty seconds is reached. Finally exhale following the same rhythm as for inhaling.

N.B.

1. INHALATION – is called. (PURAKA)
2. EXHALATION – is called (Rechaka)
3. Retention of breath is (KUMBHAKA)

Breathing control allows man on the other hand to absorb more oxygen and life force (PRANA), and on the other hand by re-establishing the equilibrium of man's positive and negative energies to bring his mental and physical states into calm, peaceful and perfect harmony.

By regular practice of complete yogic breathing and including the holding of the breath, man not only avoids problems affecting the lungs, liver, of all-bladder, stomach and heart, but can enjoy good health and vital force; this also increases the development of will-power.

To conclude, these exercises will do wonder upon one's health. In fact, when one is worried or irritated, it is advisable to go for a walk and enjoy these breathing exercises mainly rhythmic breathing.

This will make one happier and calmer. After all, it is seldom that man uses one tenth of his potential breathing capacity. Furthermore, psychologists have shown that man hardly uses one-tenth of his mental capacity. So it is quite clear that there is some connection between intake of oxygen and mental capacity. Therefore, if man increases his capacity for the intake of oxygen through breathing exercises and Pranayama exercises, his mental aptitude too would improve quite a lot. It has also been proved that slow, harmonious breathing leads to a peaceful attitude towards life. For a man who practises breathing and Pranayama exercises on a regular and timing basis, his mental control thus becomes easy.

SUPPLEMENTARY

There are also 6 types of beneficial breathing exercises for anybody and anywhere, when time is very limited.

1. Standing straight stretch out arms forwards. Take a deep breath and while retaining it, move arms sideways and again forward several times. Drop arms and exhale forcefully, widely opening the mouth.

2. Standing straight. Stretch out arms forward. Take a deep breath and while holding it, swing arms circling them like a windmill. Drop arms and exhale forcefully, widely opening the mouth:

3. Stand straight – Place fingertips on shoulders. Inhale a deep breath and while retaining it alternately join elbows on the chest and move them, wide apart several times. Exhale forcefully, widely opening the mouth.

4. Stand straight – inhale in three vigorous sniffs. On the first sniff stretch out arms forward on the second move them sideways on shoulder level on the third move them upwards. Exhale forcefully, widely opening the mouth.

5. Stand straight. Inhale a deep breath rising on the tip of your toes. Hold the breath for a few seconds while standing on toes. Exhale through nostrils keep mouth closed, while slowly lowering heels to the floor.

6. Stand straight, inhale a deep breath while raising on top of the toes and exhale while lowering the body to a squatting position then stand up.

An individual should at least go for a 20 or 30 minutes' walk everyday, either early in the morning or in the evening. Meanwhile breathing some fresh oxygen revitalizes all the organs in the body.

Position of hands and fingers:-
First before going onto comfortable sitting postures. Let first indicate the position.

60

Of the hands first.

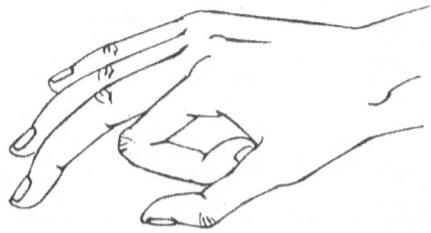

Gyana Mudra

1. Gyana Mudra (finger lock) for (Knowledge). Be in any meditation posture and fold the index fingers of both hands so that they touch the inside root of the thumbs. Spread the other three fingers of each hand so that they are slightly apart.

Then place the hands on both knees with this palm downwards and the three straight fingers, and the thumb of each hand pointing towards the floor in front of the feet.

2. **Chin Mudra** for (consciousness)
This Mudra is done in the same way as Gyana Mudra, only that the palms of both hands face upwards while resting on the knees.

One has to choose which one he is getting accustomed too.

Sitting in comfortable postures for meditation.

There are many postures or Asanas that one can get used to. But one must choose one which allows him to keep the spinal column straight and to sit easily and comfortably without twisting the legs or having any discomfort.

However, the legs and arms are not very important in meditation. What is really of fundamental importance is that the spinal column must be correctly straight.

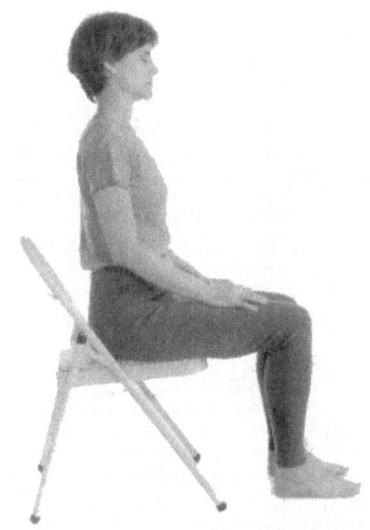

Maitri Postures

Maitri Posture chair posture: Now the easiest posture for the modern era is that one can use a chair with a straight back. This posture is called maitri asana.

One can sit comfortably on a chair or bench with the feet flat on the floor and the hands resting gently on the lap. This posture can be used by anyone, and to those who cannot sit comfortably on the floor. But remember that here as well the spine should be aligned.

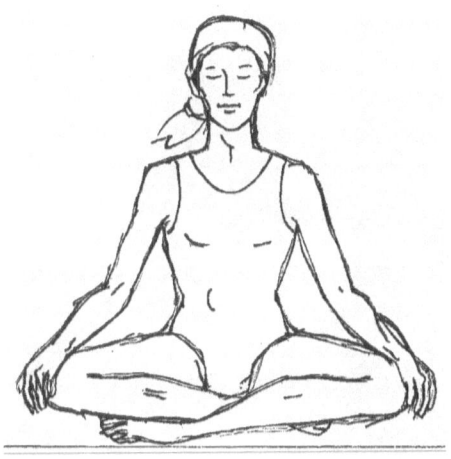

SUKHASANA

This also is an easy posture. One simply sits cross-legged as on the picture and each foot is placed on the floor under the adverse knee, and the knee rests gently on the oppose feet. One must use a thick-folded blanket, inorder that the knees and the ankles do not feel or receive too much pressure and pain.

Sit with the legs stretch in front of the body. Fold the right foot under the left thigh, then fold the left foot under the right thigh. Place the hands on the knees either in gyana or chin mudra. Finally keep the head, neck and spine straight, in one straight line.

Practise it regularly with patience, perseverence and discipline. Gradually it will become very practical and the sitting will be comfortable after a while.

PRACTICE MAKES PERFECT

Yogic Breathing
Actually this type of respiration is the way everyone should breathe. It is a combination of abdominal and thoracic or chest shoulder breathings.

Technique
The practising should be as follows:-
Inhale by expanding first the abdomen and then the chest in one slow, smooth motion until the maximum quantity of air is drawn into the lungs, then the upper shoulder. Exhale by relaxing first the upper shoulder, the chest and then the abdomen, emphasize the contraction of the abdomen muscles, so that the maximum amount of air is expelled out from the lungs.

The whole process that is from abdomen to chest, upper shoulder and from upper should chest to abdomen should be very smooth and almost like the movement of wave on the surface of the sea.

The same procedure should be followed for each exhalation and inhalation for a regular few minutes practice. After a while the process will become automatic. By this yogic breathing, one will not be easily attacked by colds, coughs and bronchitis and asthma. The vitality will improve and one will be less inclined to become easily tired. The thinking power will improve and less susceptible to anxiety or stress.

Both Yogic and Rythmic Breathing can do the boat pose for few times.

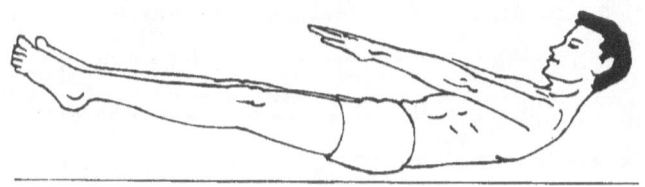

Naukasana Posture

Lie flat with back, arms at side of the body, palms facing down, inhale and raise the legs, arms, head and trunks on the same level as shown. Hold a while and exhale and return to the starting posture.

These three postures can be done on the bed before getting down the bed in the morning.

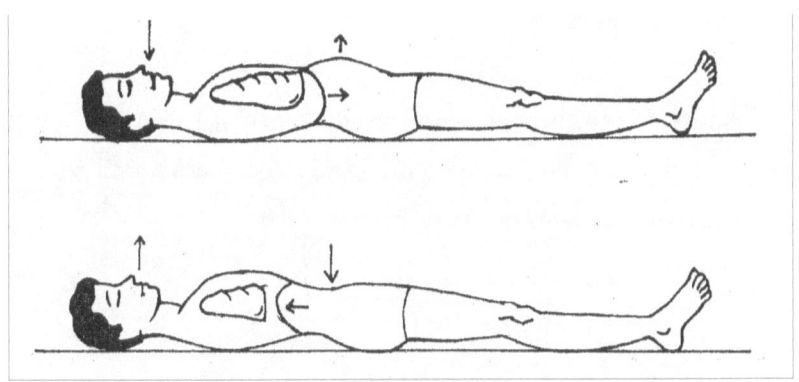

Yogic Breathing

Rhythmic Breathing

These two postures can be practised before getting in the morning, in the bed if possible. Very efficient for health as a whole.

Original and Perfect Breathing

Owing to industrialization and with a pressure of hectic living, most people even forget to breathe correctly, and they use only a small part of their lung-capacity. Therefore less oxygen is being inhale for the whole body. As you all know quite well that without oxygen life won't be able to continue, so here the breathing is shallow and the consequences are that the body and brains are starved of oxygen. However by shallow breathing, people build up stagnant air in the lower part of the lungs. Finally this lack of oxygen and incorrect respiration bring the body and mind to various diseases.

So learn to breathe properly and gain good health. Bear in mind that without breathing no one can survive.

When a baby is born, he must first breathe as soon he comes out of the mother's womb if not, no breath no life. And remember as well if someone breathes only half, he lives only half his life.

The breathing system can be divided into two processes:

1. Abdominal Breathing

One can actually have one's own experience by sitting or lying flat on one's back and placing the hand on the belly or navel. Now inhale deeply and the hand should be placed on the belly and the hand will rise as the abdomen expands. Here the diaphragm is a strong muscle membrane and it separates the lungs from the abdominal organs. The lower it goes during inhalation, the more air is inhaled into the lungs. The second movement, exhale deeply and the hand move downward as the abdomen contracts of the abdomen is stressed. Then maximum expulsion of air from the lungs will occur. During this process, do not move the chest or shoulders. Only the abdomen has the movement up and down.

Thoracic Breathing from Chest

While inhaling the chest or ribcage is expanded, in order that the ribs move outwards and upward. Then exhale and the ribs will move inward and downward. Only the chest and ribcage is in the movement, not the abdomen.

MAKARASANA

There is also a very good and comfortable Yoga posture called MAKARASANA. One will enjoy doing it definitely. MAKARASANA. Techniques or Crocodile pose. That is lie flat on the stomach and raise the head and shoulders and rest the head in the palms of the hands with the elbows on the ground. Relax the whole body and chose the eyes and breathing should be as from the abdomen not the chest. Remember well.

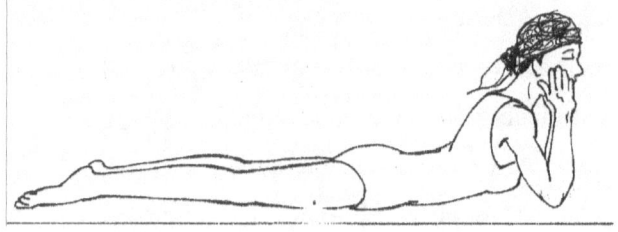

MAKRASANA (The crocodile pose)

CHAPTER 5

SURYANAMASKARA ASANA

Simple Posture I, II, III. First relax the whole body in standing posture and keep the legs apart about two feet distance or at least not together, the hands hang loosely on both sides, and the head straight. Look in front and breathe normally.

Technique and Practice:- 1st stage in a Prayer Pose.

2. Now inhale slowly and raise both hands towards the sky in a sidewise circulation movement. The time the hands reach up, complete inhaling is done. The palm should be turned forward and the arms both parallel or even one can go a bit at the back as 2nd stage. Stage III, start inhaling and bend the upper body towards the ground, keep both hands parallel to each other and move them towards the ground, in a circular motion in front. Then, by the time both hands reach near the floor, the exhaling process is finished.

Now hold the breath and remain in this posture for about 10 seconds. Keep the upper part of the body quite loose and the down part hard and rigid, the head should be between the two arms, if it is possible to put the palms on the floor or just touch the floor. But don't strain or force your body excessively, gradually and with practice, one can do the same. Be very comfortable.

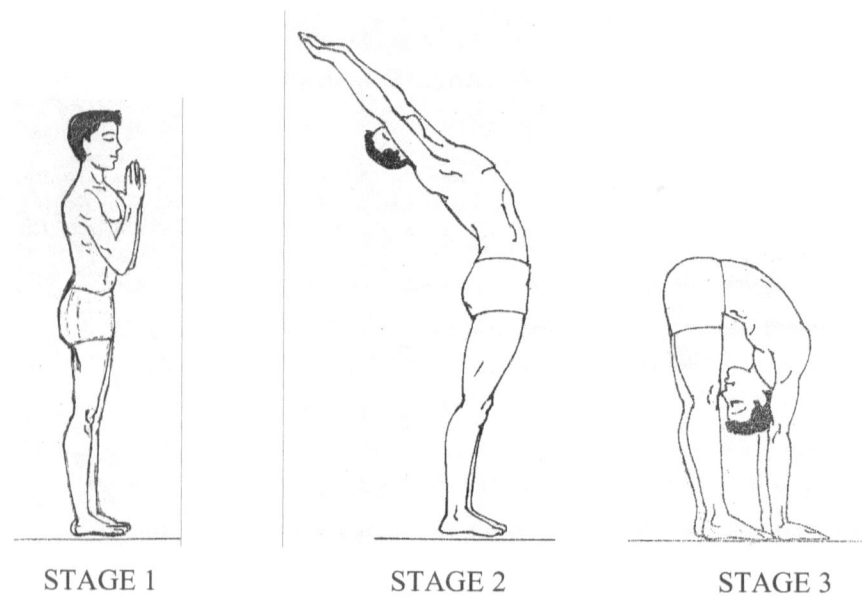

| STAGE 1 | STAGE 2 | STAGE 3 |

Finally bring both hands on the legs and inhale and return in standing position. Inhale slowly and in such a way that by the time one is returned to the standing position, one has finished inhaling. And one round of simple Saryanamask Asana has been completed. Practice one to four round every morning or more if possible.

The importance of this Asana

It activates all the glands of the endocrinal system in a mild way. It also activates the internal organs, the pancreas, adrenal, thyroid, pituitary and some other glands begin to secrete normally and their respective hormone in a normal way. As the main trouble with people of diabetic disorder results from the malfunctioning of the pancreas, the above mentioned Suryanamaskara remediates its defects by functioning it to its normality.

This asana has a good result on the stomach, spine, lungs and chest as well. Many disorders of these parts are corrected because there is a reverse circulation of the blood during performing of this asana. It also in vigorates the face tissues, the central nervous system and all the organs of the upper part of the body. It is recommended to all practitioners as it is easy to perform. Practice, persevere and be patient. The result is sure to be of great fundamental importance in one's life.

SURYANAMASKARA
WORSHIPPING TO GOD SUN
SALUTATION TO SUN

According to my own spiritual inspiration or experience, the Suryanamaskar is an asana or posture which has mysteries, which by self performing, you will be aware of these benefits. Owing to its wonderful and dynamic benefits, it is classified under the Asana exercise of yoga, and it is better to start always with this worship to sun exercise, before doing other Asanas or postures. After all, it energizes or revitalizes all the membranes and organs and system of the body, as it is a posture which covers a series of twelve physical postures on its own.

However, it eliminates all defects of sleep and it is a wonderful exercise for preparing the body and mind compound inorder the maximum benefits can be obtained from the consequent and relevant asanas, pranayama, relaxation and meditation performance etc.

Furthermore, Suryanamaskara releases and relaxes all the points of the body and meanwhile all the muscles of the body become flexing and all the internal organs get massaging. The respiratory system and circulatory blood system get activating and help to tone and stimulate all the other systems, of the body. Finally, the whole body mind complex gets harmonized and one can feel the balance and equilibrium of both the mind and body.

There is no specific preparations or time or place to perform the Suryanamaskara. Actually the magnificent time is in the morning before other Asanas are mentioned but one can practise at almost any time of the day. Whenever one feels tired, angry, depressed or tense or nervous, few rounds of this posture can be performed and one will definitely and quickly regain the loss of energy and vitality, both mentally and physically. It is also of utmost benefit, in removing emotional confusions. It is also of great pleasure to perform it because it is very symmetrical and rhythmical exercise.

My advice is, you try it and you will know what I means, it is mystical.

Now it is crystal clear, if there were no sun created by the mighty Lord, everywhere would have remained dark. Perhaps no life would have survived without the light of the SUN. It is one of the most important elements God has bequeathed to us in this universe. My experience is that there also are many suns in the total universe and it is infinity.

The word Surya means SUN plus the word NAMASKARA means either worship or salutation, so the whole posture's name is salutation to SUN or worship to the Sun.

Since time immemorial, the sun has always been worshipped and adored by ancient people throughout the world, without creed and community and colour, that is by all races. They were quite aware that the sun produces and creates the heat and light that are of fundamental importance to the nature or support of life of the universe.

Most ancient civilizations worshipped and praised the Sun in their religion and they named it by various names of God or deities. That means without sun, no life on this world, or if there is any or other planets if discovered in the future.

The sun represents spiritual illumination and wisdom of knowledge and the light in the darkness of ignorance. It also signifies the essence and the spirituality which survives in all material things on earth or anywhere. Suryanamaskar was developed as a early incoming worship of the sun, because the sun is after all, a symbol of immortality and it is supposed to die every evening and to be reborn the following morning. The rising of the sun is a moment for happiness and wonder, for it raises everything from the dead and meanwhile it reinvigorates life to everything. Many nations on this earth still pray the sun in one form or the other. Finally one can accept Suryanamaskara as an aspect of one's own regard to the sun, whether it is the material attitude or the belief in the spiritual that the material sun represents. If one is not willing to pray, then one can practise the twelve postures for the only reason to maintain and generate good health in one's daily life. This will bring to the practitioner almost a spiritual awareness, peace and harmony to his body and mind compound. This needs only to be performed a few rounds in the morning or whenever one is tired at any place.

Main Characteristics
Suryanamaskara constitutes five important features. The practiser must perform all of them in a methodical way to derive the best favourable outcome.

The five characteristics are
1. Body postures
2. Breathing
3. Mantras
4. Awareness
5. Relaxation
1. Body postures-Asanas:- There are twelve postures which conform to the symbols of the zodiac.
2. Breathing – The three actions of inhalation, exhalation and retention of breath should be practised together with the corresponding twelve postures. Without following the breath and

the movement, many of the main advantages of Suryanamaskar are left out.

3. Mantras – Very important. There is a specific mantra corresponding to the twelve postures in Suryanamaskar. When performing the twelve postures, a respected mantra is uttered either silently or loudly with each posture. The combination of specific breathing and mantras energizes the entire mind and intellect. And the advantage when uttering the mantras loudly and devotionally can cure an ailment or can acquire stability of the mind and self-control or dispersing the tensions and stress occurred by modern way of living.

The twelve mantras in chronological order are given here:-
1. Om Mitraya Namah – Friend
2. Om Ravaye Namah – Shining
3. Om Surya Ya Namah – Beautiful light
4. Om Bhanave Namah – Brilliant
5. Om Khagaya Namah – Who moves in the sky
6. Om Pushne Namah – Giver of strength
7. Om Hiranyagarbhaya Namah – Golden centered
8. Om Marichaye Namah – Lord of the Dawn
9. Om Adityaya Namah – Soul of Adith
10. Om Savitre Namah – Beneficient
11. Om Arkaraya Namah – Energy
12. Om Bhaskaraya namah – Leading to enlightenment

4. Awareness :- This a very fundamental love of the Surya Namaskara, if there is no awareness one will not gain the maximum advantage

5. Relaxation:- This is a very separate posture which one must do without failure in ending the twelve postures. Actually the very best method is Dead posture, Shavasana. A separate chapter is deals with it, refer to chapter IV.

Rounds – How many:-

Actually this depends on the stamina, health and the time available. One should do it easily and in a relaxed manner, not till one gets tired. Beginner, one or two rounds and gradually adds more rounds. If one is reasonably in good health, one can perform up to twelve rounds in the morning. If one is doing more asanas, this should be done in the beginning as it helps to remove any sleepiness and relaxes the body in preparing for other asanas practice. And the best time to do Suryanamaskara is during morning and at sunrise, while facing the sun one can absorb the health by getting the ultraviolet rays from the sun. It should be practised in the open air, in the lawn or a clean flat surface. A blanket can be placed on the ground or floor. It can be performed at other time during the day and after 3 hours after the meals. Whenever one feels tired, tense or unrest during the day, few rounds can be done as relaxing remedies. Finally some mental effort is needed to memorize the various positions, breathing and the mantras. One may need the instructions to be read from friend while performing suryanamaskara. A guide or teacher (Guru) is of most fundamental importance for the beginner.

The benefits one derives from Suryanamaskara are enormous. It brings the systems and organs of the body such as circulatory, digestive, elimination, respiratory, endoctrine, nervous, muscle skeleton and subtle influence into equilibrium and balance with one and another and meanwhile helping to prevent and eradicate diseases.

To conclude, there is no reason why man cannot perform it daily. There is no exercise that can beat it. I do recommend one to practise and see it for oneself. No doubt that running, swimming and walking are very good exercises; unfortunately they don't give complete benefits exercise and energy such as Suryanamaskara. If one does not want to practise other ASANAS but at least try one's own level best to perform Suryanamaskara daily in the morning. It requires only a few minutes and the body will be fully balanced and get complete energy to carry on during the whole day positively and one can face all sorts of daily difficulties of the modern life of tension and stress. This exercise is recommended to anybody, either in cities or suburbs and from everywhere in the world. It is an elixir for our modern dreadful life.

Now the technique of the 12 postures with breathing guide or mantras. First get used to breathing systems while practising and when the habit is formed, then repeat the mantras together while breathing and performing these postures:-

After executing these recommended Asanas and Postures, I recommend people to have at least 20 minutes of walk daily in the morning and evening if possible, if not at least 20 minutes in the morning which is of fundamental benefit for daily health.

Either one believes it or not, just for curiosity, try it for God's sake for your inner self. May God bless you all.

Now Position I Begin

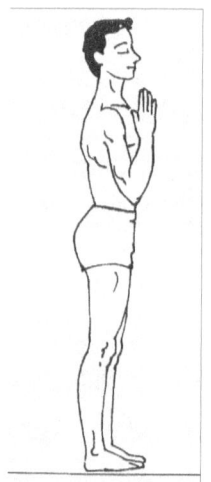

PRANAMASANA

Position: No.1 Prayer Pose – Exhale

Mantra: Om Mitraya Namaha, Salutations to the friends of all.

Concentration: Heart center

Chakra: Anahata

Maintain your awareness

Stand straight with feet together. Place both palms together in front of the chest and exhale fully, the pressure of the palms and the effect of this mudra on the chest area.

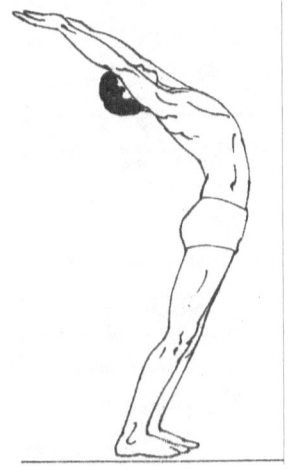

HASTA UTTANASANA

Position: No.2 Raised arms pose, inhale

Mantra: Om Ravaye Namaha, Salutation to the shining one.

Concentration: Neck Center

Chakra: Vishuddhi

Raise and stretch both arms above the head with palms facing upwards. Arch or bend the back and stretch the whole body. Inhale while moving into position, stretch the head as for back as in a comfortably as possible and be aware of the curve of the upper back.

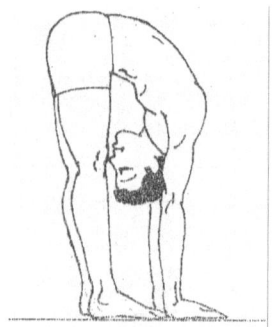

PADAHASTASANA

Position No.3 Hand to foot pose, exhale.

Mantra: OM Suryaya Namaha,. Salutations to he who indules activity

Concentration: Root of Spinal Column

Chakra: Swadhis Thana.

The movement continues bend forward from the hips. Bring the hands to the floor on either side of the feet and the head as close as possible to the knees. Legs straight the breath in exhaled while moving into position. The back should be kept straight. Concentrate the awareness at the pelvis the pivoting point for the stretch of the back and leg muscles.

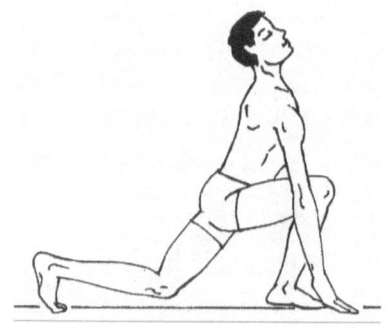

ASHWA SANCHALANASANA

Position No.4 The equestrian pose: Inhale.

Mantra: Om Bhanave Namaha, Salutations to He who illumines.

Concentration: Eyebron Center

Chakra: Ajna

Keeping both hands in place, one either side of the feet, bend the right knee while extending the legs backwards as far as possible. The right toes and knee touch the floor. Bring the pelvis forward, arch the spine and look up. The Fingertips touch the floor and balance the body. The breath is inhaled while bringing the chest forward and up. Focus your awareness at the eyebrow center. Feel the stretch from the thigh moving upward along the front of the body till the eyebrow center.

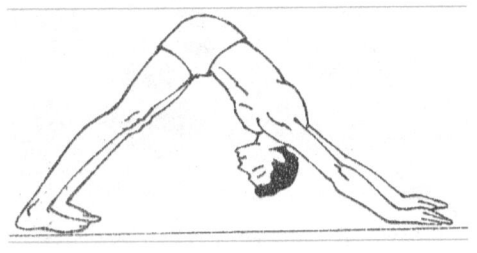

PARVATASANA

PARVATASANA

Position: No.5, Mountain Pose. Exhale.

Mantra: Om Khagaya Namaha, Salutations to the one who moves through the sky.

Concentration: Neck Center

Chakras: Vishuddhi Dddhi

Bring the left foot back and place it beside the right simultaneously raise the buttocks and lower the head between the arms, so that the body forms a triangle with the floor. Exhale while doing the movement. Aim to put heels flat on the floor. Bend the head as far forward. So that the eyes are looking at the knees. Focus awareness on neck.

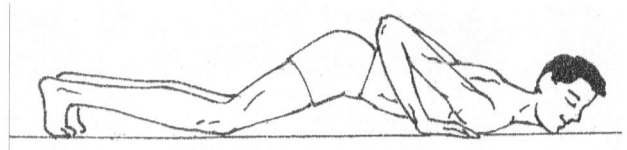

ASHTANGA NAMASKARA

Position: No.6. Salutation with eight limns

Mantra: Om Pushne Namaha, Salutations to the giver of strength and nourishment.

Concentration: Behind navel.

Chakras: Manipurakha

Bend the knees to the floor and bring the chest and chin to the floor as well, keep buttocks elevated. The hands, chin, chest, knees, and toes touch the floor and spine is arched. The breath is retained in exhalation from position 5. This is the only time that the alternate inhalation and exhalation of the breath is changed. Awareness focused at the center of the body or back muscles.

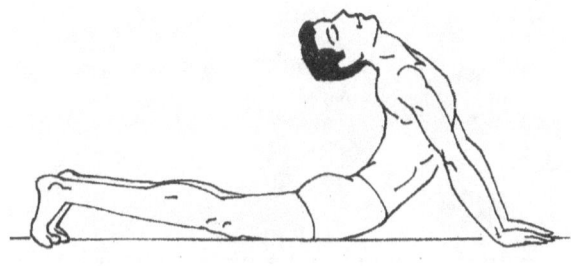

BHUJANGASANA

Position: No.7 Serpent pose: Inhale.

Mantra: Om Hiranyagarbhaya namaha, Salutations to the golden cosmic-self.

Concentration: Root of Spinal Column.

Chakra: Swadhisthana

Lower the hips while pushing the chest forward and upward with the arms until the spine is fully arched and the head is facing upwards. The legs and lower abdomen remain on the floor and the arms support the chest upward. Inhale moving forward and upward. Awareness is focused at the base of the spine feeling the tension from the forward and upward. Awareness is focused at the base of the spine feeling the tension from the forward soul.

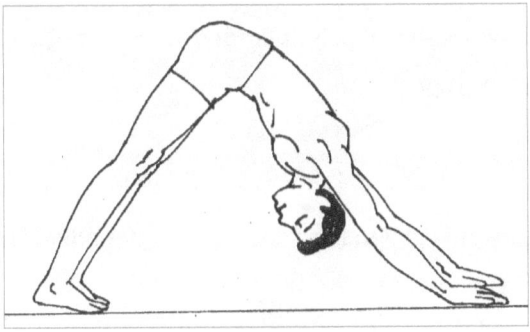

PARVATASANA

Position: No.8 Mountain Pose: Exhale.

Mantra: Om Marichaye Namaha, Salutations to the rays of the sun.

Concentration: Neck Center.

Chakra: Vishuddhi.

Keep the arms and legs straight while pivoting from shoulders, raise the buttocks and bring the head down to restart No.5. Exhale while moving to position.

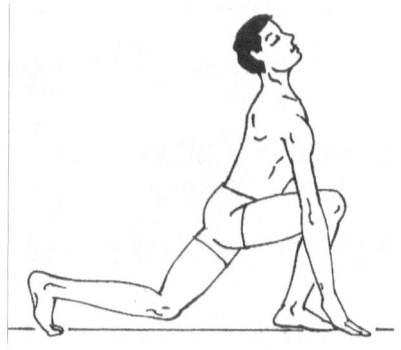

ASHWA SANCHALANASANA

Position: Equestrian Pose, Inhale.

Mantra: Om Adityaya Namaha, Salutations to the sun of Adiji.

Concentration: Eyebrow Centre.

Chakra:- Ajna.

Bring left leg forward, placing the foot between the hands simultaneously bring the right knee down to the floor and pelvis forward. Arch the spine and look up to restart No.4. Inhale while moving into the position.

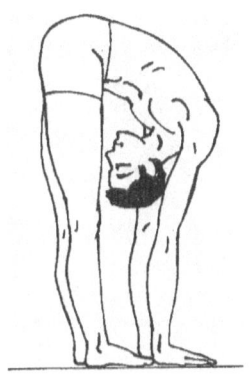

PADAHASTASANA

Position: No.10 : Hand to foot Pose. Exhale.

Mantra: Om Savitre Namaha, Salutations to the stimulating power of the sun.

Concentration: Root of Spinal Column.

Chakra: Swadhisthana.

Bring the right foot in beside the straightening the legs, bend forward and raise the bullocks while bringing the head in towards the knees. Hands remain on the floor beside the feet back to the posture No.3. Exhale back to the posture No.3. Exhale while moving.

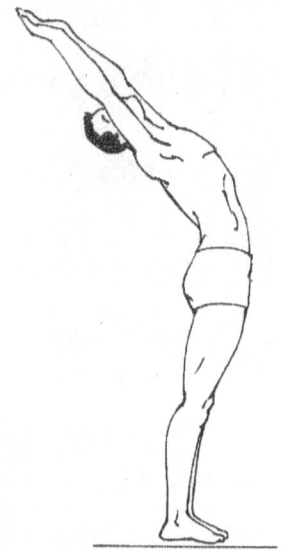

HASTA UTTANASANA

Position:- Raised arms posture: Inhale.

Mantra: Om Arkaya, Salutation to he who is fit to be praised.

Cocentration: Neck Center.

Chakra: Vishuddhi.

Raise the torso, stretching the arms above the head. FLEX back wards to resume posture 2. Inhale in this moving position.

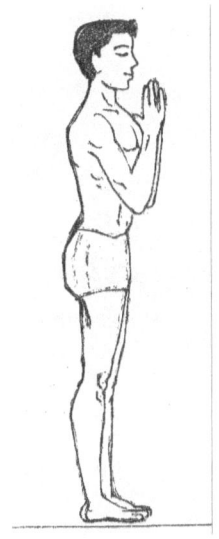

PRANAMASANA

Position: Prayer posture. Exhale.

Mantra: Om bhaskaraya namaha, Salutations to the one who leads to enlightenment.

Concentration: Heart Centre.

Chakra: Anahata.

The body straight and bring the hands together in front of the chest, Back to Posture 1. Exhale. Then relax half round of Suryanamaskara is completed.

This makes half a round of the Surya Namaskara i.e. first part now to constitute the other half round, the same procedure is needed; the only change is that the left leg is brought back in posture 4, and the right leg moved forward in pose 9. So one full round is completed and it contains 24 movements of 2 sets of 12 postures. When completing this, give a balance to each side of the body in each half round.

When the 12 postures are completed, inhale while lowering the hands on both sides and then relax, then start the second half round of the practice with exhalation. If you feel tired on the first half round, you can rest taking full breath, inhalation, exhalation and inhalation before starting again the second half round.

There should be full awareness of body and postures. Ask the question. How do I feel? And be comfortable and assure that the breath is slow and relaxed.

CHAPTER 6

NERVOUSNESS AND RELAXATION

Nervousness is the opposite of calmness, tranquillity and relaxation. It is after all a pair of the situation in one's body. But we do not realize this, as people very frequently ignore these situations, and the consequences are that they think that they are sick and ill by the occurrence of symptoms within the body. So they feel or believe that they are ill and look for remedies, visiting doctors, whereas they can, indeed, control these situations and get cured by relaxing or calming their own mind.

The root of uneasiness springs or germinates in the mind itself. It happens because when external or internal problems cause anxiety, worries or uneasiness in the brain of a person, his normal behaviour and functioning of the mind becomes disturbed, which in turn affects also the normal situation of the body. Here it is noticed that the factors which produce anxieties, worries and uneasiness are also the cause of nervousness at the same time. Now if the duration is short and momentary, it can be remedied immediately, but if it becomes prolonged, eventually it not only affects the health and poise of the person, but his role, behaviour, thoughts, actions, moods and the whole of his normal way of life. In this hectic modern world, therefore, it is of fundamental importance for men and women to know about it and how they can get it controlled and at the same time get it cured by relaxation techniques and methods.

However, nervousness creates many symptoms in the person in different ways. A person who is nervous can be easily recognized by his countenance, his body language and his behavioural aspect. So, it is very difficult for a nervous person to be at ease, relaxed and attentive. Nothing is soothing and pleasant to him. Mistakes crop upon his common habit. He gets fed up very soon. And finally he loses his sense of balance and equilibrium and the default is reflected in almost everything he tries to perform in his daily work and life. He is also very absent-minded.

What are the aspects, situations and factors that cause nervousness:- There are three main categories but I am not going to describe them into detail as you are acquainted with them.

1. Environmental Aspects.
2. Social Aspects.
3. Personal Aspects.

1. Environmental aspects are those which happen due to the pecularities of natural phenomena. These are natural calamities such as earthquake, drought, famine, flood, hurricane, epidemic and etc, etc. These might bring enormous anxiety, worry and due to the fear or safety or loss of property and disturbances in the situation of life.
2. Social aspects are situations such as feeling of economic insecurity, in finding out a decent job, career and profession, social disturbances due to religious conflicts, ethnic, racial and political tensions and conflicts, fear of war and many other problems in this

modern world, all created by man only, inorder to lead a satisfactory and material life. Unfortunately the contrary is often the case. Frustrations, disappointments and disillusions are causing strain, distress and restlessness; in spite of people's extreme effort, they are incapable of true happiness and mental peace. Thus under such situations and circumstances, definitely nervousness is the price paid.

3. Personal Aspects. Under this aspect, there are countless factors, but only these four basic factors are considered here.

1. Feeling of Fear.
2. Lack of proper understanding of human nature and social phenomena.
3. Feeling of hurting others.
4. Problems about sex life.

Nervousness would be eliminated with the acquisition of proper knowledge by the individual himself and not by anybody else.

Vivekananada says:

"All the knowledge that we have in this world, where does it come from? It is within us. What knowledge is outside? No knowledge is in matter; it is in man all the time. Nobody ever creates knowledge: Man brings it from within."

When man's mental peace is unconsciously or consciously shattered or broken or disturbed, the balance is also broken and shattered and then any misfortunate can occur.

Thus, the science of yoga says;" "Know this balance, cultivate this quality of balance and act, think and live according to the same principle of balance. It is no use going to extremes. Try to keep a balanced life, which means neither too much indulgence nor complete abstinence"

Yoga means and advises a normal life when possible.

Food:-
1. One must have good quality food but not quantity.
2. Physical exercises. Few minutes regular practice of Yoga asanas, pranayama, rhythmic breathing, relaxation, concentration in one's daily life.

Nervousness remedy:
1. Deep breathing.

This deep breathing will have a very beneficial effect on the nerves. Nervousness will be alleviated, if not completely removed. One can practise it at any place, in office, in travelling and home, no matter the stomach being empty or full. Use it whenever you need it.

Techniques:-
Be seated or in standing position, one can be seated in chair, sofa, or on floor. One should sit in a straight up manner, keeping the spine and head straight or if one is standing be straight.

Then exhale all the air through both nostrils; after the air is thrown out, start inhaling through both nostrils. Take a deep breath. When inhaling is completed, then start exhaling. Continue this process for about ten rounds. While exhaling and inhaling, be in a slow and steady way. Do not do deep breathing, rest for a minute or more.

This will render immediate relief to the individual of his nervousness. Try it for your own.

Before ending, my advice is that most of the time, the mind is the chief factor for good or ill, of the human body. Diseases in the human body are caused by mental tiredness and unrest very often. Since this is true, treating the body wisely proves benefic. "Physicians are learning now that they cannot adequately treat the body unless they treat the mind as well."

Even doctors have scientifically proved that even ulcers, arthritis and other body symptoms can originate in the mind, due to such emotions as fear, envy, lost, anger, jealously, uneasiness, anxiety, worry, jealousy and so on, this is called psychosomatic.

So next, one should relax, as in relaxation, the mind and body are in a calm soothing, restful and comfortable condition.

RELAXATION

In our modern era, most people are nervous, worried, stressed or depressed because of the daily pressure and hectic life of this modern, material and so-called civilized world. So the mind becomes clogged with fear, anxiety, worries, so one is no longer able to enjoy a robust and normal mental health. All these problems are happening because modern man works in a hurry, loves in quick way, eats in a very fast manner and even rests in a hurried way. Eventually, one is too much busy and the art of marvellous relaxation and meditation is definitely forgotten and even unaware of. Therefore, owing to the unrestful and unrelaxed life, all sorts of neurasthenia, sleeplessness, cardio-vascular troubles, indigestion, constipation, headaches and lots of other diseases have become frequent and prevalent among modern individuals.

People cannot adequately treat the body, unless they treat the mind as well. Most people in a busy city are tense and strained with fears, worries, anxieties and frustrations appearing on their faces. Here, the very importance of relaxation should be underscored, as every individual should make it a must to follow the routine and regular discipline of the relaxation techniques in life. Then one will remain in a harmonious, calm and peaceful state within oneself.

The question, however is asked, what is relaxation? Relaxation is a situation when the individual, I mean the individual himself, is in a complete restfulness. The individual himself is not tense and is at a complete easiness. Remember that both the body and mind are in a comfortable position, resting calm and tranquil. In fact, when an individual is completely relaxed, then he really enjoys the restful moment and can have the needful sleep during the night. Here what I mean is that, if one is being relaxed, one is having a proper rest and sleep, which in another way means one is leading with the proper life-force, energy, vigour and power for a satisfactory and pleasing mental and physical life style during the next day. The amount of work and pleasure really very much depends on our state of "RELAXATION".

Owing to the fast developing world, most men and women in nearly every culture and community cannot at all feel restful and relaxed. They are tired, uneasy and restless and in the end, they become nervous, so they can hardly have a proper sleep. It all happens because of the troublesome situation of this modern and hectic age. Man seems reluctant to rest and relax and with their feverish living, they become helpless and unable to rest and relaxed. There is no sad spectacle as to see people addicted to drugs such as sleeping-tablets and alcohol. Finally, this leads to various harmful and injurious things to themselves, ignorantly by taking these pills to get some sleep.

These tablets are mere palliatives and may cause a lot of harm to the body and mind. And by the time one realizes this, an incurable damage has already been done to the body and mind.

In our hectic pace of living, it is a matter of fundamental concern for modern humans to be aware of what relaxation is, what causes people to be tense and what are the remedies. Here through yogic methods, man can have a proper knowledge and awareness of these vital aspects. These can also enable man to acquire a satisfactory and proper knowledge of curing the body and mind from their disturbances.

Unrelaxed symptoms: – Owing to lack of relaxation, several identifiable changes in the healthy condition of the individual are noticeable. The individuals themselves can better detect and feel these changes within themselves. Then the sure remedy will be easier. The symptoms are as follows:- forgetfulness, lack of alertness and cheerfulness, lethargic performing of mental work without habitual efficiency, getting fatigue quickly, a haggard look dullness in appearance and activities, lack of habitual charm, grace and brightness in the face etc..

Causes of unrelaxed individual:-

There are many factors in an individual's life that can make him restless, factors such as various social, environmental and personal aspects. There factors have already been explained under the topic of nervousness. Owing to social environmental and personal reasons, anxiety is caused in the individual and the major problem it does, is to make the individual unrelaxed. When restlessness becomes chronic, nervousness gnaws at the root of the individual. However, one can say that lack of relaxation is the beginning stage of such nervousness.

There are also people who cannot rest or relax and sleep properly due to some mistakes they have made previously in their preferences in choosing the wrong actions and possessions in their daily life. And they have no proper knowledge of certain essentials of relaxation. Bear in mind as well that lack of relaxation in one individual might affect the relaxation of another. However, the individual must have a proper understanding of his external and internal character as a whole. There are also many foods and drinks that cause restlessness to people. They are coffee, tea, tobacco and smoking. Taking too much or abusing these things may be harmful to the individual's health. There are also certain other factors which might also cause restlessness such as eating hot meals, over-eating, excitation, writing or reading provoking and sensual books, magazines and other materials before going to bed, listening to exciting and sensual music, participating in passionate and lustful conversation with friends etc.

The individual should pay attention to certain importance inorder to have a proper relaxation. They are proper condition of the body, place, bed and environment during the time of relaxation. So a proper attention to things in individual daily uses are as important for relaxation.

Yoga way of Relaxation

From the Yogic point of view, the individual must first have a deep understanding of himself, the social environment and his physical and personal factors. And secondly he must have a self-controlled character and determination of correcting and changing his previous bad habits which have been caused by an ignorant way of living. This can be done by determination and willingness on the part of the individual alone. No one can do this for him "HE IS HIS OWN DESTINY AND FATE."

It is crystal clear that when some one is hungry, he himself has to eat and his stomach will be definitely filled up. No one can eat for him. From the scientific point of view, doctors prescribe drugs to individual to relax. This is only momentary and besides drugs leave lots of side effects to the human body and brain in the end. How is it possible for medicine to correct anxiety, lack of understanding, bad habits, manners, like and dislikes in an unrelaxed individual?

The individual is himself responsible for his own bad or better health of his own body and mind, and a relaxed temperament during the whole day.

The yogic way is of two means: first to correct doing certain things and second of practising some postures as (SADHANA)

FOOD:
To be relaxed, one should eat plainly cooked food and without too much spices. One should not consume hot stuff, too much salt and pepper, hard, fried, roasted and dry food. One can have soft liquid or juicy food.

Food should be taken at least two hours before retiring to bed. The most important thing is that the stomach should not be heavy, and it should not be stuffed at the time of rest and sleep. In any case, if one feels thirsty or hungry at bed time, a little juice or pure water can be drunk, but not solid food of any kind. Take only one or two cups of coffee or tea within twenty four hours. By all means, one must have a balanced diet in one's daily life. After all equilibrium in everything is needed for a proper living. So here the Science of Yoga brings is a good balance in one's life and this leads one to spiritualism.

1. Smoking or Cigarettes. It is a great killer of humans. The individual thinks that he is having a good relaxation by smoking, but ignorantly, he is poisoning himself. See how far it damages the lungs internally.

   If in case one is a smoker, smoke hours before retiring to bed; however, if one cannot stop smoking, at least cut it to the minimum in one's life. It is one of the killer-drugs. Smoke addiction is very harmful as the lungs are the most important organ in a body, because without air, there would not have anything which can move in this universe.

Reading before retiring. Many people have the habit of reading before going to bed. Never read such books and magazines which excite and arouse sensual feelings or provoking one's lust. Instead if one wants to read, then read such books which can provide one with relaxed feelings and make one jovial before retiring. Read books such as short stories, poems, books of wild life and of natural beauty and comics; better read scripture and spiritual ones, of which we have a wide literature.

Now the body and mind conditions are the most important in life. First, it is crystal clear that one's body must be hygienically clean before going to bed. One must take a hot or cold bath or shower once a day; this also depends upon the temperament of the individual and the climates. After all, one has to adjust oneself to one's way of living. Everyone has his own way of living and free to live as one likes, but without discipline, one's life is a misfit and miserable. Remember well that the body is the ship and mind is the captain of the ship, both have equal importance to reach one's destination in daily life. Furthermore one must clean the mouth, teeth, eyes, hands and the feet while going to sleep. If one has a shower or hot bath or a wash to hip, one must wipe out the water with a dry towel before going to bed; this would be very helpful to sleep peacefully and at the same time have a good relaxing sleep during the night. Secondly, the mental condition should be kept free from worries, anxieties and the problems of day to day life when one is retiring to bed. There is a method which is not so easy for everyone to do it, but it is only a very important suggestion if applied by anyone.

This method is that before retiring, one should sit for ten to fifteen minutes. First take paper and pen and jot down all things one needs to do on the next day. Read them once more carefully and plan or memorize the works for the next day, then go to bed without any worry about daily problems. By applying this method at least the mind will be relieved.

Now if in case one has problems of long range nature, make another list and same thing should be done as well; note down the things one will need in the month to come and what one intends to do in the coming future to tackle the problems of life.

Some useful disciplines:-

One should have a routine to sleep. Avoid changing habits or hours of sleep. Most important the bed must be free from bugs and dirt, it must be pleasant and clean and not too soft as well. Don't allow any noise to penetrate into the room while going to retire. Unless one has a liking for keeping the lights on, switch then off. Before going to sleep, put off the music as well.

While going to bed, just lie down comfortably, have complete rest and no thought for sleep. This must take about ten to fifteen minutes or may be more for getting actual sleep. These last minutes are critical for conditioning the body for sleeping. Thus, one should not be concerned with any problem. However, when the mind, body nerves and muscles are being relaxed and at complete rest for a while, then one can only expect to have a sound and peaceful sleep.

Then these above disciplinary measures are enough to provide one with full relaxation. If inspite of all the disciplinary measures, one still have some difficulties in relaxation, then one has to follow the Yoga posture. SHAVASANA: Relaxation Posture.

YOGA METHOD OR RELAXATION

Meanwhile, this regular practice of simple relaxation posture will make it likely for one to learn to let go and to eject negative thoughts from one's mind in the same way that one turns off the lights when they irritate one's eyes.

However, merely by reading the written words won't do one any good or bring one anywhere. I do stress heartfully that in practising, persevering and patience that one can get the truth of it. Why don't try to execute the relax posture fervently and with confidence and properly right now? This will take one only a few minutes and the result will certainly be positive for one's own good forever and ever.

Never forget that one who learns to relax, learns the secret of a successful and healthy living with a long and easy life.

Technique SHAVASANA – Sleeping or death Posture.
The Position to start.
To start with, take off heavy dress, always be in T-shirt or short or in very loose and light dress. Glasses should be put aside. Lie on a carpet or spread a heavy bed sheet or cover. Lie down on your back, keeping the whole body loose and in a straight position, your palms should be on the floor on both sides and open upward. No pillow should be used. Eyes should be kept close and the whole body should be on the floor in a complete relaxed way.

In this posture, you are ready to start and stay in this situation during the actual practice.

Ready to Start

1. This is a very good relaxing therapy for the eyes and mouth as well. your eyes should remain close for two seconds. Then open them for two seconds, carry on the opening and closing of the eyes for at least four times. Now the eyes open again look upward then downward and straight. Then look first towards left and then right. Then straight again and lastly close the eyes again. Continue this eye- exercise for three to four times and stop. Now the mouth should be opened wide without any restrain. Then turn the tongue inside the mouth in a way that the tip is folded back towards the area of the throat and close the mouth. The mouth closed and the tongue fold for 10 seconds. Now while opening the mouth, bring the tongue back to the normal situation and close the mouth again. Continue this exercise for three to four rounds.

2. After having performed all the eyes and mouth exercise, now keep your eyes closed and concentrate on the tip of your toes and see that the toes are relaxed. Mentally imagine and move slowly upward and towards the head by verifying what you feel; legs, knees, thighs, waist, spinal cord, back, shoulders, neck, arms, palms, fingers and all the area of the body are actually very relaxed. Finally you can feel that your body is completely relaxed. As you are relaxed, now think that your body is getting heavier and heavier. So heavy that it sinks into the carpet etc.. and you no longer feel its weight. Stay like this for a few minutes, completely relaxed and at ease and feel yourself light.

3. While relaxing the body, now relax the mind with this following process. Choose a view of natural beauty which you have ever visited and loved, such as a garden or a river side or a green place of mountain etc.. and feel as if yo are present mentally at that scene. This time fix your vision to that place and feel as if you are part of this place and enjoying the scene and breathing the air of the same surrounding. While your mind is involved in the scenery surrounding, practise some deep breathing. While doing deep breathing slowly and the rhythm of the stomach should go according to the breathing up and down, inhaling and exhaling. Slowly make about ten to twelve rounds. When the deep breathing is complete, think as if you are feeling sleepy. Now you are really completely relaxed, then stay in this situation for ten minutes. You must feel and enjoy the relaxing moment.

Finally move all you head, hands, wrist, fingers, legs, feet and toes both sides, right to left smoothly and have a deep breathing, then open your eyes and stretch your body and then be seated and stand up and do a little massage all over your body. That means, you have completed the relaxation posture.

One can do this before going to bed or early in the morning when all exercise and postures are over. To conclude, if one continues to practise this everyday, one will be able to get rid of one's tension and cast off one's worries, laziness and anxieties at will.

May The Lord The Almighty Be With You. For the caring of your own mind and body which are two weapons of your daily life and to take you to your destination.

SITTING AT ANY EASY POSTURE ON A CHAIR OR SLEEPING POSTURE, RELAX PROCEEDURE SAME.

RELAXATION – BODY AND MIND CONTROL
9. SHAVASANA (Dead Posture)

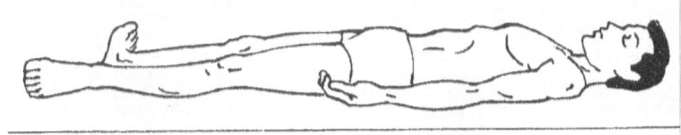

1. **Starting Position**: Complete Relaxation. First thing lie down on the back. Keep the body straight and completely loose. The palms both sides and should be upwards. The breathing should be normal. Let the whole body lie on the floor in our unrestrained way. The eyes should be closed lightly. This position be maintained throughout the practice.

The technique now:-
1. Close the eyes for two second. Then open than for two seconds. Practise this opening and closing of the eyes for at least three to 5 times.

2. Now open the eyes again and look upwards and downward, then straight. Now look toward the left and then towards the right side, then straight again then close the eyes. Do this eyes exercise for two or three times.

3. This time open the mouth wide without strain. Then turn the tongue inside the month in such a way that the tips of the tongue is folded back towards the throat area after close the month. Keep the month closed for 10 seconds. Then open the mouth and bring the tongue back to its normal position in the month. Do this for two or three rounds.

4. Now keep the eyes closed and bring the mental attention towards the toes. Mentally see that the toes are complex loose and relaxed. Then again mentally move slowly upward towards the head area by checking and feeling the knees, thighs, waist, spinal cord, back, shoulders, neck, arms, palms, fingers and rest of the areas of the body to be sure that they are actually relaxed. Make a slight move of the neck and head by turning right and left. Then the head should rest in a comfortable position. Now one will feel that the whole body is physically relaxed.

5. Finally relax the mind as well with the following process. Now choose a place of natural beauty which one has ever witnessed or visited and attracted by it. For example a part life garden, a river side or a sea side etc.. and feel as if one is mentally present at that beautify and vivid view or place. Feel as if you are lying at that place really and breathing the air of the same environment. Now while keeping the mind involved with that plan do some deep

breathing. In this deep breathing, just inhale and exhale slowly, but deeply. Remember that during the deep breathing the stomach should go upward while inhaling and in should go downward while exhaling. Exhaling and inhaling make one round. Do it slowly and smoothly not quick process. Make about 10 round of them when the breathing is over, feel as if the sensation of going to sleep. Now completely relax and stay in this position for ten minutes. Then after open the eyes and stretch the body and then come the in the sitting position. Don't get up immediately. Then the SHAVASANA is completed.

This is one way of doing Shavasanas relaxation. But there are many ways of performing Shavasanas.

I am herewith introducing a second position one can choose any of them which one is preferred:- This also is complete RELAXATION.

First before going to MEDITATION, it is of great benefit to practise a concentrated relaxation posture exercise. Actually this one relaxes the whole body muscles and gets rid of any fatigue or strain and it also energizes both the body and the mind as well. While performing this posture, keep the mind alert and concentrate on the breath as one progressively relaxes the muscles. In the beginning, practice only for 5 minutes and gradually one can go up to 10 minutes, not more as the mind will begin to wander and may feel oneself drifting toward sleep.

Once one has a complete control and get used to it, then one may proceed to longer period.

The technique

Put oneself in the dead posture with the eyes slightly closed. Inhale and exhale through the nostrils slowly and smoothly and deeply without any strain. Remember that there should be no noise, jerks, or pauses in the breath. The inhalation and the exhalation should flow naturally, with exertion in one continuous movements. Keep the body loose and still.

Now mentally travel through the body and relax the top of the head, forehead, eyebrows the space between the eyebrows, eyes, eyelids, cheeks and nose. The exhale and inhale completely four times, breathing diaphragmatically.

Exhale, relax the month, jaw, chin, neck, shoulders, upper arms, lower arms, wrist, hands, fingers and finger tips. Feel as if one is inhaling form the fingertips, up the arms shoulders, face to the nostrils and then exhaling back to the fingertips. Then exhale and inhale completely four times.

Relax the fingertips, fingers, hands, wrists, lower arms, upper arms, shoulders, upper back and chest. Concentrate at the center of the chest and exhale and inhale completely four times.

Relax the stomach, abdomen, lower back, hips, thighs, knees, calves, ankles, feet and toes. Exhale as though the whole body is exhaling and inhale, as though the whole body is inhaling. Now, expel all the tension, worries and anxieties. Inhale vital energy, peace and relax. Exhale and inhale completely four times.

Relax the toes, feet, ankles, calves, thighs, knees, hips, lower back, abdomen stomach and chest. Concentrate at the center of the chest, exhale and inhale completely 4 times.

Relax the upper back shoulders, upper arms, lower arms, wrists, hands, fingers and fingertips, then exhale and inhale completely 4 times. Relax the fingertips, fingers, hands wrists, lower arms, upper arms shoulders, neck, chin, jaw, mouth and nostrils. Then exhale and inhale completely 4 times.

Relax your cheeks, eyelids, eyes, eyebrows, the space between the eyebrows, forehead and tip of the head.

Finally allow the mind to be aware of the calm and serene and peaceful flow of the breath for 30 to 60 seconds. Let the mind make a gentle, conscious effort to guide the breath so that it remains smooth, calm, and deep without any noise or jerks.

Now, gently and smoothly open the eyes, stretch the body. Try to keep the calmness, peaceful feeling throughout the day.

This one is my favourite before going to bed and whenever one is tired or exhausted.

SITTING ERECT – SUKHASANA:-

Sit in an erect position as in the meditation posture. SUKHASANA. Let the whole body rest or become still. Relax the muscles of the chest, lower back, and abdomen while maintaining an erect posture.

Now observe the flow of the breathing and practise the yogic breathing. Up to 4 times. After finishing the process then move to the relaxation of each part of the body from frontal head to the toes.

First relax the frontal head, eyebrows, eyes, cheeks, nostril, lips, chin, neck. Then relax the shoulder joints, upper arms, elbows, lower arms, wrist, hands, fingers and finger tips, now form finger tips to fingers, hands, wrists, lower arms, elbows, upper arms then shoulder, shoulders joints.

Now, relax the chest cardiac cavity, stomach, navel, belly, then, lower part, hips girdles, thigh, knees, calves, ankles, feet and toes. Then the second part with the same procedure from the bottom toes up to the frontal head is done in the same above mentioned ways. So when the frontal head is reached breath 4 times and feel that the whole body, head are completely relax and finally repeat the pranava mantras. Om 5 times and shanti 3 times and end the relaxation session, don't raise immediately rest for at 30 seconds, then move up and try to be in this relaxation feeling throughout the whole day.

After days of practice regularly morning and night, one will be really out of anxieties and stress. Always use one's right mental attitude, the results of one past Karma, that one will have to suffer. Do not worry or alarm oneself about this. If calamity does befall, accept it. Think constructively but do not ponder or brood on the same. Finally this will not hurt or affect one in this whole life. If one has secured the higher form of consciousness, nothing will harm him. But if one is superstitious and fearful, one's instructive mind might accept these harmful thought waves. It is all the condition of one's mind, believe me or not.

If anything goes wrong, do not blame others. Blame oneself alone. Change one Karma through virtuous actions as well honest thoughts and holy words which do not hurt others. It is only a Guru and saint that can change Karma or the bad Karma can be changed or forgiven.

Swami Vivekananada says:-
Stand up, be bold, be strong, take the whole responsibility on one's own shoulder, and know that one is the creator of one's own destiny. All the strength and succour one wants is within oneself. Therefore one's own future depends with good action and control mind, senses, and satvic food (pure) while performing Yoga in the daily life to attain higher spiritual level.

"NEVER HURT OTHERS or never give any heart-pain to others, for you will only hurt yourself."

Remember Buddha's sayings:
"If a man foolishly does me wrong, I will return to him the protection of my ungrudging love, the more evil comes from him, the more good shall

go from me, the fragrance of goodness always comes to me, and the harmful air of evil goes to him."

After all, we are all here due to our past Karma and we are here on this earth to perform our task and do our duty without hope of reward. As Krishna has said in "GITA".

Now I end up with my personal experience. If one practises the relaxation technique, one will feel that one's mental attitude has changed definitely. I have not consciously tried to change my mental attitude. It has changed gradually and automatically with the practice of these above techniques. This is called the mystery of the Science of yoga.

So here by controlling the mind by the technique of the science of yoga, definitely the mental attitude is changed to the better condition.

I have here described a few yoga steps such as Shrasanas, relaxations, postures and descriptions, it is up to you to choose your favourite ones.

There should be practice, patience, perseverance and discipline. And finally this world with be definitely a better one to live in. If not, to my dismay, the world will be going from bad to worse. Pray God that this does not happen to the coming generations

THE SCIENCE OF YOGA IS THE ONLY SOLUTION
A REMEDY TO THIS MATERIAL WORLD

CHAPTER 7

CONCENTRATION

"You are what you think as well," goes a saying. The great Rishis, Swamis and genuine mystics have brought to mankind the eight steps of the Astanga Yoga. These will definitely help humans to attain the purification of the body, mind and soul, finally to reach union with the Supreme Being or to wake up from his sleeping and immanent.

The eight-fold steps are:

1. Yama (control and discipline, self-restraint).
2. Niyama (Rules, methods and principles)
3. Asanas (making body postures)
4. Pranayama (kryas with air and the real process of rhythmic breathing)
5. Pratyahara (Avoidance of unpleasant or harmful actions e.g knowing the proper actions)
6. Dharana (Concentration on which I lay more emphasis).
7. Dyana (Meditation)
8. Samadhi (Contemplation) Reaching the level of superconsciousness.

These are being described in the end of the chapter. So concentration is the sixth step of the Astanga Yoga. It is classified under the RAJA YOGA and is the first step before proceeding to meditation and contemplation. From my spiritual inspiration, meditation is too high for ordinary human beings as are much people involved in the material fake world (Maya). So here concentration and relaxation are beneficial paths to follow for humans in the modern era.

When referring to history, one will learn and come to know that by intense concentration, there have been always geniuses, such as the blind poet Milton, Shakespeare, Einstein, Newton, A.Fleming and Gandhi etc..

Here concentration means the one-pointedness of the mind according to the great will-power of the individual. So, it is crystal clear that by producing or revealing this will-power which is really inside every individual that the individual becomes master of his own mind and definitely controls its instabilities and weaknesses. The individual can command his mind and also his body to be in harmony, peace and calmness. His mind does wonder and attach itself to countless issues, undesirable thoughts, objects and events. When concentration is practised, the mind becomes very selective in some necessary purposes. Unnecessary and worthless attachment and desire are cut off.

When proper training and discipline of concentration is followed, it definitely has a complete curative result over the problems of sickness and the mental disorder; which most of the modern people are suffering unknowingly from such as compulsive obsessive disorder affecting quite a number of people. Don't forget that the nature of the mind also affects the nature of the body. So here there is an interrelationship between the mind and the body.

Here, it is said, "You are what you think. You are what you eat, and you are what you breathe."

So, to lead a very jovial and peaceful living, there should be a balanced in mind conducive to a healthy and disciplined body. Then the individual will reach his true destination towards Godhead, the Almighty. After all, we are all here in the human incarnation to attain or reach Him. But owing to this illusionary world, we do forget our true nature and we return to the cycle of birth and death.

I don't want to go into much detail, but I am giving a hint and clue on how to follow the ways and how to practise CONCENTRATION. Its preparation and disciplines are of fundamental importance in every individual's life; then the miserable problems of one's life will be definitely avoided. One can detach and stay very calm and peaceful and free from mental sickness or problems (whatever you call it).

To start with, one should have a very good interest and wilfulness in the practise of concentration. Furthermore, the object on which one has chosen to concentrate must be there, materially or mentally. There can be no concentration without a noticeable degree of INTEREST and ATTENTION shown by the aspirant.

One has to create interest and then there will be attention. This means that interest develops or creates attention. Both should go together, then there will really be good positive concentration.

If the object is very interesting, then there will be great attention. When one is doing concentration, one must plunge oneself in it. Forget oneself and be lost in the Self. Shut out all other thoughts and do one thing only; do not to think of any other things and thoughts. Remove duality and be one-pointedness and then concentration will become easy and the goal will be definitely reached.

However, an attentive man can only develop his will-power with a combination of interest, application and discipline, then this can work mysteries, keeping the balance of mind in minus and plus, that is remaining the neutral, this is real wisdom. And if one is able to practise this, it is really a wealthy man in this world, though he may be a clad in loin cloth, ill-fed, ill-housed. He will be very robust in will-power and mind though he has a very weak physical body. "He eats only to live, but not as the so-called modern man of material belief, live to eat."

Worldly material human beings have lost their balance in the pursuit of trivial and frivolous actions. They become very irritated and often lose their temper quickly. Imagine how much energy, life-force (PRANA) is being wasted unnecessarily in one's daily life by indulging in such materialistic and the off-sung secular interests.

Those who want to develop a proper balance of mind and body should develop detachment, discrimination and be a fervent practiser of CONCENTRATION. Control and concentration of mind is very difficult but not impossible.

Try, try, try till success comes. Remember that you are being made from the five elements water, fire, air, earth and ether, so everything is within you. Bring out the latent power and it is the right time for you all to attain the goal. Man is the microcosm of the macrocosm.

Lord Jesus says:-

"EMPTY THYSELF, I WILL FILL THEE" Don't forget that Man is a complex social animal. He possesses circulation of blood, digestion system, respiration, nervous system and excretion system as well ete, etc... He has thinking, perception, memory, imagination. He also thinks, sees, tastes, smells and feels. So spiritually speaking, he is the image of God, that means God is within. But he is ignorant because he has lost his divine glory by eating the forbidden fruit, the allegory of Adam and Eve of the Bible. By mental discipline and practising the Yoga of concentration, he can gain back his lost divinity.

N.B: Scientifically talking, it is no advice to eat meat, fish, eggs, spices, curry, fried food and even snacks and soft green drinks etc, but people are going against the rules of his body only to satisfy their uncontrolled senses.

FEW CONCENTRATION TECHNIQUES
1. TRATAKA – KRIYA OR CONCENTRATION

Trataka means steady gazing. The practice of trataka involves gazing at a point or object without blinking the eyes. It is a method of focusing the

117

eyes and turning the mind on one point to the exclusion of all other objects or concepts. (one-pointedness)

It falls under Hatha Yoga in which there are six way of purification, which are called Shatkarmas and Trataka is the sixth step of the types of yogic purification done by the eyes (outer gazing). Trataka is of fundamental importance as in a sense, it acts as the bridge between Hatha Yoga and Raja Yoga.

1. Technique:-
Keep a candle flame in front of you and try to concentrate on the flame. When you are tired of doing this, close your eyes and try to visualize the flame. Do it for half a minute and increase the time from five to ten minutes according to your taste, temperament and capacity. You are not required to force your eyes to stretch them to the fullest extent, they have only to be kept open in a natural way. The muscles around the eyes should not be stretched. You should not wear glasses and if you have an eye problem, don't practice Trataka. You must learn it from a Guru or a knowledgeable person.

2. Technique
This is my favourite one and very easy to perform.
Sit in your favourite posture about one foot from the watch. Concentrate on the tik-tik or tik-tok sound of a clock slowly. Whenever the mind runs, again and again try to hear the sound. Just see how long the mind can be fixed continuously on the sound.

3. Technique

One can do so by fixing a flower, such as (Rose) afterwards a picture (photo) of your favourite saints, statue or deity. First sit in any relaxed postures. Make the body straight. Head, neck and the spine should be in one line and straight up, and do not tighten it, make it loose. The breath should be normal. Now ready to begin the practice of concentration (DHARANA), the first step is controlling the wavering of the mind.

Now, start looking at the flower petals. Keep looking for about ten to fifteen seconds. In case you feel pain in the eyes, close the eyes for a short time. Try not to blink the eyes. When having looked at the flower for ten seconds, then close your eyes gently and try to vision the shape of the flower in your mind. Let the eyes close for about ten seconds, while you are trying to recall the image and shape of the flower in your mind. After keeping the eyes closed for ten seconds, open them and again look at the flower for another ten seconds. Repeat the same procedure a few times, that is seeing through the eyes, closing the eyes and then seeing through the Inner eye.

Repeat this procedure only five times in one session during the first week. Gradually develop it up to ten, fifteen times, which should remain as the limit. If you practise ten times only in one session, that will be sufficient. But in no case should one go beyond fifteen times in a single session.

When the practice is done, keep sitting still. Now loosen the body and sit in a relaxed way for two minutes, then it is over. After that, you are free to eat, sleep or do any work.

After two months, you can change and practise with some photos, statues of your own liking. These should be of medium size, bright colour which are soothing and pleasing.

1. Christians can do it with a photo of Christ.
2. Muslims can do it with photo of the wording of ALLAH.
3. Hindus with photo of KRISHNA (which I recommend) and others according to their liking and tastes

ARRANGING POSITION

N.B.: Keep the flower or photo etc.. in the same level with the eyes in the sitting position. The flower should be about one to three feet in front of the sitting place.

All my Blessing and Love to you all "MAY THY LORD SHOWER HIS GRACE UPON YOU ALL."

The Sage Patanjali introduced these yoga to worldly people to get out of this miserable stress which is an enemy to worldly man nowadays.

HATHA OR ASTANGA YOGA

In all my books you will find that I do stress immensely on Astanga and Hatha Yoga which has the eight limbs or folds within it. Through these yoga, man can reach his spiritual level and meanwhile can reveal his innerself by practicing fervently and regularly. So by sincere practice one can be completely aware of the Raja Yog gyan Yog, Karma Yog and Bhakti Yog. If one gets this complete awareness of the above mentioned, no one can stop him to reveal his inner Guru and can definitely get the guidance of a true enlightened Guru in the only human form even by living in this material world.

So I am enlightening the Hatha Yoga which was introduced by the great Sage and Yogi, Patanjali at that ancient time. He forecast the yoga practises to relieve the modern evolution and material man from his difficulties from modern STRESS in his daily living.

Yoga practice is the only discipline to reach perfect stability. But a Guru is of a great help, without Him no one can attain the highest spiritual level, whatsoever practice is done. He is the gateway to God as he is Himself God. I know it is hard but not impossible. It is all to the individual undertaking and daily practice of the real path of the Yoga Science and art of real living.

Remember that common or ordinary people can practise Hatha or Astanga Yoga which includes the eight limbs or folds that is Yama, Niyama, Asana, Pranayama, Pratgahara, Dharana, Dhyana and Samadhi. One can definitely attain Karma, Bhakti, Gyan and Raja Yoga after educating this power, they can reach the highest destination of liberation (Moksha) self-realisation God and if they go beyond, then, there is no return to reincarnation of the circle of birth and death. One becomes PARAMATMA or

121

PARABRAMAH, the only stage of which God wants all of us, humans to reach in this species, but unfortunately all people get themselves entangle in the Maya world of unreality. They don't want to know themselves and for them reality is unreality and the unreality is reality they get always control by the enslave of illusionary world..

To the great sage Pantanjali, the eight fold steps are as follows:

1. YAMAS

Yamas = self restraint. They are five in this stage of Yamas.

1. Ahimsa = (non violence) That is not to do any injury to living being through thoughts, words and deeds. One must love the entire creation, non-violent. This Ahimsa has been a core teaching of the Gandhian philosophy.

2. Satya = That is truthfulness, to say exactly what one sees with one's own eyes, hears with one's own ears and understands through one's own brain. It means that truthfulness should not only be external, but internal as well.

3. Asteya = That is not to steal anything and not to be tempted by the lustful enjoyments through thoughts, words and deeds.

4. Brahmacharya = keep one's sense organs including the organs of procreation under control and not to be tempted by the lustful enjoyments through thoughts, words and deeds.

5. Aparigraha = That means non-covetousness of users. In Asteya, one may accept charity, but not to steal. But in this one, even charity is also not accepted. Hoarding of wealth, riches and other materials of enjoyment for selfish ends is Parigraha, while the absence of this is Aparigraha.

122

The practitioners have to follow sincerely these rules and to continue on the second one, which is Niyamas.

2. NIYAMAS:- This also has five rules:

1. Saucha = That means purity external and internal. The purity of mind is especially to be stressed. The body can be kept clean and pure by Satvic food, six types of Yogic purifications etc.. Mind purity is achieved through giving up of all attachment, jealousy and other vile ideas inorder that the disciple's thinking becomes clean and pure.

2. Santosha = That is contentment. A disciple should be content with whatever is gained while doing one's duty truthfully or whatever is received through the grace of the Almighty.

3. Tapas = that is keeping the mind detached and under control and bear pleasure and pain, heat and cold, hunger and thirst with equanimity.

4. Swadhyaya = That is to study spiritual books to acquire real knowledge and to spend one's precious moment in the company of good people, sages and exchanging ideas with them.

5. Ishwara pranidhana = That is complete surrender of self to God in words, deeds and thoughts; it is practice of the non-ego. That is to worship God, chanting His glorious name (Japa) hearing about Him and thinking of Him as all-pervasive, omni-present and omniscient.

After the disciple has done the upper practice with sincerity and devotion, now he can follow the ASANA, body postures at the same time.

3. ASANAS

A daily regular practice of Asanas is a must for keeping the body fit and the mind pure. These asanas have been described as sitting in a comfortable posture, the body straight and firm. To transmit a state of effortlessness to the body, to do away with all the effects of over-indulgence of body in worldly affairs and to give it a necessary rest is the object of these asanas.

A regular practice of these Asanas results in the purification of veins and arteries and nerves and to promote general well-being.

Now the most important as well is the Pranayama, that is this breathing system of the respiratory organ.

4. PRANAYAMA:

Pranayama means here of controlling the normal breathing cycle. As already much stressed upon, pranayama aids one to get rid of worldly desires and sensual drives and thereby it leads to knowledge. Ignorance that covers the knowledge is removed. Mind becomes easy of concentrating and the evils are burnt by practising Pranayama. When sushumna is activated by practising pranayama, it influences the whole nervous system, thereby developing latent powers of man. And these powers are also named Siddhis, through which miracles can be done.

But remember that yoga is practised to make one realize one's innerself, not to do miracles and make money for name and fame.

Actually people compare PRANA with air or breath and therefore describe Pranayama as the exercise of breathing. This is a very misleading and a wrong conception, because PRANA in fact is the vital energy or life force which pervades each and every element of the world, whether organic or inorganic. This is a cosmic force throughout the whole hemisphere. It no doubt refers to the air and breath.

But remember well that PRANA is not only the air, it is the vital energy in the air. While talking of Pranayama, one should always bear in mind the difference between the air and the vital energy within it, the meaning of Pranayama is the expansion of prana. The purpose of Pranamaya is to inspire, control, infuse, regulate and balance the PRANA SHAKTI in the human body.

Pranayama purifies the mind, improves power of concentration and leads to sound mind and body.

5. PRATYAHARA:- That means the withdrawal of these senses from their specific outsided objects and projecting them inward. The senses are wholly turbulent and restless. Practising Pratyahara brings the senses under control, imparts to the body health and capability to enter superconscious state.

Through the practice of these four first parts :-Yamas, Niyama, Asana and Pranayama, the body becomes pure and healthy, mind and senses are more restrained and in harmony. In fact, it is easy for one to achieve concentration. One starts to get a glimpse of the powers of the Almighty and gets merging oneself into Him. All these developments and achievements prepare the ground for Pratyahara.

The great Yoga master, Patanjali, has highlighted Pratyahara in the five external organs of Yoga, that is Yama, Niyama, Asana, Pranayama and Pratyahara. Finally Dharana, Dhyana and Samadhi are its internal organs.

6. DHARANA, Concentration

This is to fix one's mind on an external object, subtle or otherwise, like hearts, Lotus, nose or one's favourite deity this is called Dharana. After practising the five stages, Pratyhara brings the mind and the senses under control, so once the mind is at peace, it can then concentrate successfully on any object. Remember that when concentration is performed in a state of delusion it does not achieve its destination.

A boat without oars cannot reach its destination. Dharana without the oars of consciousness cannot lead one across to the ocean of life. By practising Dharana, freedom is achieved from the cycle of death and birth and meanwhile all one's woes disappear. One should practise it daily and regulate the food, thoughts, words and deeds to reach perfection.

126

7. DHYANA

Here meditating with constant attention on the object of concentrating is Dhyana. Any evil tendency can be erased by Dhyana and not through any other means. Dhyana purifies the mind of Rajas and Tamas gunas and lights the mind with satvic gunas. Actually Dhyana should be done for twenty four hours, not only to sit for few minutes only. That is the true meditation.

8. SAMADI – Super-Consciousness

This is the eight and last stage. This is the state of superconsciousness and perfect calm. When the mind becomes one with the form of the object in Dhyana, this leads to the state of Samadhi.

It is the culmination of Dhyana, when Dhyana reaches maturity, the mind loses the sense of duality with the object of concentration. Dhyana leads to the state of samadhi. The disciple has to practise Dhyana in it fullest form to reach this highest stage.

In Dhyana, the object of Dhyana, the self who practices Dharana and Dhyana itself appears to be separate and different from each other. But in the state of Samadhi, the only thing left is the object of Dhyana, because all the three becomes one in Samadhi, the difference between the self and the object completely disappears; the One in all and the all in One of the mystics.

These three are collective and when one achieves maturity, the intellect is fixed on this only. This helps to unfold the world of knowledge and wisdom to the disciple and reaches superconscious state. "The well-resolved mind is single and one-pointed, but the purposes of the irritate mind are many branches and endless," the Geeta enjoins.

CONCENTRATION – DHARANA

Before proceeding on Dharana CONCENTRATION, I want to stress that everything goes into pairs, Negative and Positive, good and bad, plus and minus, macro and micro, animate and inanimate, male and female, it goes like this etc, etc the ying and yang of the Chinese. Even in the human form, one has left and right as well and by Yogic point of view even man and woman must have this two X + Y within themselves, if not nothing will workout. This is duality, the relativity of Einstein.

So here what I mean is that one must have discrimination within oneself and furthermore one must know how to surrender oneself. These two are within the human being.

For example, if one does not surrender before going to bed, he will never fall asleep. And if one does not discriminate, then one can even eat his own feaces as one can witness this in animal.

However, one has a mind and body and the one which one does feel and see is the ATMA "Soul," so by thinking only God and by doing good action and feed the brain and body with SATWIC food and qualities, then one can have the presence of God within oneself.

Now by doing concentration for a few minutes either in morning, midday or evening, one can take the road to Spirituality.

First to have a good concentration, one must have a remarkable degree of interest and attention. These two should work together, without interest and attention, no concentration is possible.

Remember that all the great writers and Scientists must have interest and attention, then they can accomplish their inventions or their creative works. So with these two, they can concentrate and reach to one-pointedness.

Concentration is purely a mental process and one must use it for self or God realisation. Human is an intricate and intelligent social animal. He can use the art of reasoning and have an art of living and is a biological organism. He is also characterised by the belongings of certain physiological functions such as an organic system and body physiology as blood circulation, digestion, respiration, excretion and brain etc..

He also has the possession of character, knowledge of wisdom and especially of certain phychological functions as thinking, perception, memory, imagination and so on. Actually he can see, think, taste, smell and feel. Spiritually and philosophically viewing, human is the image of God and may say that he is God himself.

However, by not using his discrimination and with surrendering himself to the material slavery world, he has lost his Divine glory ignorantly by becoming a complete slave to this illusionary and material world. Take for example Adam in the Bible he lost his divinity by tasting the fruit of the forbidden tree. And the Demon has become blind by using the ego of power in accumulating name and fame. Human can regain his lost divinity by mental discipline and the Sadhana of the Science of Yoga, such as the practice of concentration, relaxation, postures, asanas, pranayama and meditation. Man has only to snatch and devote a few minutes out of his precious 24 hours and definitely he will reach his goal toward his inner self, his inner world, his Essence.

Finally concentration, Dharana, is a complete cure for all our mental disturbances. As the mind is focused on a constructive principle, uneasiness, restlessness, worry, anxiety, the attitude of self-depreciation all these maladies are banished out of the body system.

After all, concentration does not depend upon how much time spent, but on how well one holds oneself together. As one is able to co-ordinate one's body, one's mind and all one's scattered forces and succeed in making them as one, one realizes in full measure one's innate efficiency.

Concentration gives power and it implies great self-control of mind. A true concentration is strength, that is strength of mind, of character and cannot be used for destructive purposes or to satisfy personal desires. By concentration, one obtains stability of the mind. Concentration means effort. It also means overcoming physical and mental habits. Mental strength can overcome physical habits, but mental habits are more difficult to control. The mind always can help one to overcome physical tendencies. If the mind is strong enough and the desire sufficiently one-pointed i.e well concentrated, even inveterate, such as drinking alcohol and the drug habit can be conquered through the one-pointed mind.

KRISHNA has said:

"As a lamp placed in a windless spot does not flicker, the same smile is used to define a Yogi of subdued mind practising union with the self."

"When the mind is completely subdued by the practice of Yoga, and has attained serenity in that state, seeing SELF by the SELF, he is satisfied in the self alone."

Concentration is an ability of body, mind and soul. There is a physical concentration and there is mental concentration. The first one means gathering together every ounce of bodily strength and directing it one-pointedly; the second is more difficult but gives unlimited power to the mind and by constant practice, it is possible. To end here, "as a man thinks all in his heart so is he."

CONCENTRATION TECHNIQUES

1. Sit on a chair straight or in a favourable ASANA posture about one foot from a watch clock. Concentrate on the tik tik sound slowly. Whenever the mind runs, again and again try to hear the sound. Just see how long the mind can be fixed continuously on the sound.

131

2. Sit in front of a candle flame in front of you and try to concentrate on the flame. The flame should be two to three feet distance. When your eyes are tired of doing this, close your eyes and try to visualize the flame. Start for half a minute and increase the time gradually to five minutes. It should be performed according to one's taste, temperament and ability.

3. One can fix either on a black spot or on one's own deity picture. Fix the eyes on the above mentioned till tears come in the eyes or the eyes start burning, close the eyes and visualize the black spot or the deity picture. One can practise as from 30 seconds till five minutes. This also according to one's taste, temperament and capacity. These techniques have been clearly discriped above on concentration TRATAKA.

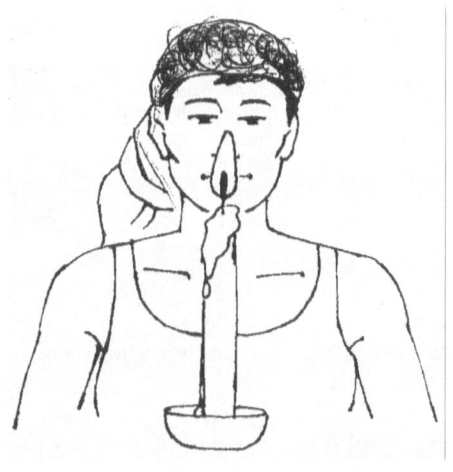

TRATAKA
Don't forget that practice makes perfect.

CHAPTER 8
MEDITATION - DYANA

Meditation is the seventh step in the Science of Yoga. Meditation is first to sit still in any yoga sitting posture and relax the whole body. Secondly, control of breath and mind, these two work together, that is the breath should be balanced and the mind one-pointedness, thirdly comes concentration on one's objects only and then finally the fourth is meditation when one is completely absorbed in the SELF.

"Perfection in meditation comes from perseverance and devotion to the Supreme," Patanjali opines.

If one wants to follow any spiritual path, one must become well aware of the fundamental righteous disciplines, such as non-injuring, non stealing, truthfulness, continence, external and internal purification, contentment, control of the senses, detachment, discrimination, self-surrender to and study of the scriptures. One must not give way to jealousy, anger, hatred or unkindness by thought, word or action. One must not crave or envy; one must speak the truth fearlessly and observe chastity, inner and outer cleanliness and self-restraint, and faithful in one's higher study, and in devotion to one ideal. Until these disciplines are firmly practised and fulfilled, no amount of outer practice can help one.

Remember that if one has anything material in one's life but which is at variance with spiritual disciplines, no amount of sitting still and trying to meditate will bring one this blessing of contemplation.

One who has not good control over one's body is unable to make proper use of one's mind, one can never concentrate much less can one meditate. It is clear that if the mind is not balanced, one cannot sit still even for a few moments. Therefore, the maintaining of posture is to acquire firmness of both mind and body. Finally, one who lacks mastery over either one's physical or mental organism cannot gain spiritual consciousness.

Breath is next to be considered because breath is life itself. Through breathing the life-force or life current (Prana) flows into all parts of human body and mind. It is that Prana which sustains the whole life in humans. This fundamental truth has to be repeated.

In our feverish modern tempo and the acceleration of information Technology, people don't get time to think and derive the proper benefit from the breathing systems. Because with the stressful and fast way of living, one does not know how to regulate one's breath. Actually, one breathes automatically, involuntarily and unconsciously, but one must learn to breathe consciously and properly and rhythmically.PRANAYAMA, rythmic breathing etc.. is the controlling of life-force to common control of the breath. By controlling the breath, one can fill oneself with vital energy and thus eliminate all the physical and mental defilements.

Finally, cultivate the habit of faithful practice with discipline, regularity and perseverance. One must create a divine principle within oneself. It is all internally and nowhere or no one can do or give you this divine power. One must create it. Chist says:- "If therefore this eye be single the whole body shall be full of light."

KRISHNA says: "When the mind is completely subdued by the practice of YOGA and has attained severity, in that state, seeing Self by the SELF, he is satisfied in the Self Alone."

Meditation changes one's mental attitude and opens the gate of the mind to intuitive knowledge and many powers. One can get whatever one wants and the worldly thoughts are shut out from the mind.

Now, meditation is of two sorts. 1. SAGUNA (with Gunas or qualities) meditation and 2. NIRGURA (without gunas or qualities) meditation.

SAGUNA is the method of Bhaktas, that is meditation on Lord KRISHNA, Jesus, Rama, Shiva etc… It is done with form and attributes or qualities.

2. NIRGUNA – This a method of Vedantine. This is done on the reality of the SELF. Meditation on mantra. Om Soham, Allah, Amine, Amen etc…..

It is concentrating and meditation that ultimately lead to SELF-REALISATION or GOD REALISATION.

Meditation is a particular technique for resting the mind and reaching a state of consciousness, which is above from the normal waking phase but not excluding the latter. When in meditation, one is fully alert and awake, but the mind is not centered on material world or on the events that are taking place all around the meditator.

However, the mind is not asleep, dreaming or fantasizing. On the contrary, the mind is clear, relaxed and centered inwardly about the SELF.

Meditation is a therapeutic system to the body and mind from time immemorial. It helps relaxing the muscular tension and the self- activating nervous system and relieves the whole body from mental stress. A person with a meditation attitude has a peaceful mind and his immune system by reducing its reaction to stress and strain. Meditation also diminishes one's need for sleep and energizes one's body and mind. Meditation is simply a process of quiet, effortless, one-pointed centered of attention and awareness.

Finally, in meditation, one simply observes the mind and let it be calm and quiet, allowing one's mantra to lead one deeper within, by exploring and experiencing the shallow level of one's being. But meditation is not a religion. Meditation is a mode of life that requires not one to change one's beliefs, reject one's culture or change one's religion. True meditation is not concerned with any religion at all. On the other hand, it is a practical, scientific and systematic technique for knowing oneself in all our aspects.

It has nothing to do with the institutional structures of the world, but is a clear and simple method of discovering the inner dimension of life and finally by setting up oneself in one's own true nature. Religion instructs man what to believe, but meditation teaches one how to experience directly for oneself. No conflict should be done between these two approaches.

Meditation should be practised with purity, and with a systematic and orderly structure.

To meditate one will need to learn:-
1. How to relax the body
2. How to sit in a postural and steady position.
3. How to change one's breathing system (Pranayama) rhythmic breathing natural and undisturbed and peaceful.
4. How to observe peacefully the objects powering in one's mind without any rest.
5. How to discriminate the good thoughts and bad thoughts and at the same time to learn to accept those which are positive and helpful to one's spiritual growth in living; that is within 24 hours for your own sake, find out this precious time to know yourself, to communicate with your own reality, that is the SELF. Then one can really come to know the almighty God. He is WITHIN US ALL.
6. How to stay fixed and unperturbed in any situation, whether be bad or good.
7. Before one meditates, give 3 to 4 hrs after having a big or heavy meal.

8. Study carefully what one has eaten and how it affects one's meditation after in the day.

9. One should be careful and must select fresh, wholesome, easy digesting foods which foster the clarity, calmness, vitality and energy to meditation.

Believe me, that one has to do the practice and find out for himself. This is self-practice; no one can give you or do it for you. You are your own responsibility and you have all this divine power which is dormant within you. Please awake it as you are the only race of humanity that can realize this.

Human is the only creature who can execute it and no other living and non-living thing can do this. You have the precious birth to be born as a human being, don't retrograde or fall backward. Reach your destination (God) and GOD ONLY.

My blessing to you all who want to follow the path to perfection or divinity.

Thus to end here, the orderly process of practising is the following:-

First – Bathing or preparation.

Second – Stretching exercise or yoga postures.

Third – Relaxation exercise.

Fourth – Breathing practices.

Fifth – Concentration and the finally

Sixth – The meditation process itself.

By now, hoping that you have been well informed and ready to go into earnest practice. One need not go to forest or mountain or an ashram. One can still carry out with one's own daily works and duty, but must find few minutes in one's every day life, that is within the 24 hours for one's own sake to find out this precious time to know oneself, to communicate with one's own reality, that is The SELF. Then one can really come to know the almighty (God). HE IS WITHIN US ALL.

Don't believe blindly. Don't look for God in other humans or in animate or inanimate things. You yourself have the potentiality to find HIM first within yourself; practise the innerquest and conquest.

How you can know the taste of the food, if you have never tasted the food yourself for your own experience. Don't use other's experience. Do it yourself. Then you will know the TRUTH AND ONLY THE TRUTH. HARI OM TAT SAT.

Now a few techniques will be described. You can practise them or you can approach a real master to learn them, from him and persevere in the method he gives you till the end.

What are needed are discipline, regularity, perseverance, determination, faith and sincerity to surrender inorder to reach that destination.

Remember Buddha says:-

1. "To suffer from yourselves, none else compels. None other holds you that you live and die. And whirl upon the wheel and hug and kiss its spoke of agony. All the misery and trouble one has is of one's own choosing. Such is one's nature."

1. **Techniques:-**

This is a very easy practical meditation on OM. (PRANAVA).

Do practise this morning, midday and evening or at least during morning and night.

Repeat 21 times Om, starts from your navel to the throat and finally to Sakasrara top of the head, the highest CHAKRAS

1st five times Om – For 5 Outside INDRIYAS.

2nd five times Om – For 5 inside INDRIYAS.

3rd five times Om – For the 5 KOSAS.

4th Five times Om – For 5 elements and finally

6th One time Om - For the ATMA that is the 21st and last time. Then rest.

Or one can do as much Omkar if one has enough time to do it.

2. **Techniques**

Sit on Padmasana or Siddhasana or Sukhesana in the meditation chamber. First thing is to relax the whole body and make the mind very calm. Then watch the flow of the breath very silently. One will hear the sound of the inhalation and exhalation, the sound made is "SOHUM" that is "SO" during inhalation and "HUM" during exhalation. The meaning of SOHUM is I AM HE OR HE AND I are the same. After a while, one will feel and remind the breath as one's identity with the SUPREME SOUL. Actually

140

one is unconsciously repeating SOHUM 21600 times daily at the rate of 15 SOHUMS per minute. While practising the Sohum meditation associate the ideas of existence, knowledge, bliss, Absolute, Purity, Peace, Perfection, Infinite and Love etc... Negate the Body and Mind complex while repeating the Mantra and identify oneself with the Atman or the Supreme Soul.

3. Techniques:-

Concentrate and meditate on the infinite blue sky. This is another kind of Nirguna meditation. By concentrating, the mind will cease thinking of finite forms. It will slowly begin to melt in the ocean of Bliss, as it is deprived of its contents. This mind will become subtle and subtler.

Finally one can create one's own way of meditation as I have said, we are all our own creators. For once you see God within, then you can see Him in anything and anywhere. After all, we are part and parcel of HIM. Either you believe it or not. But a trial is always worth trying for one's own belief. Here, to `see' is with the inward eye, "other than the known and above the unknown."

CHAPTER 9
DIET means Balanced Diet
FOOD – YOU ARE WHAT YOU EAT
THREE CATEGORIES OF HUMAN FOOD

In yoga, food plays an important part in an individual's daily life. Food is an obligation to the individual's spiritual, mental and physical growth from womb to tomb. Whether in Yoga, Science or medicinal term, food is the origin of vitality in an individual's life. However, any improper food intake will definitely bring disorders of any type in the human body. That's why one should have a very good awareness of the proportion and quality of the food that one usually eats in daily life.

Yoga has described food into three different grades and classes, so that one might be very vigilant in one's daily diet throughout one's life.

1. 1st class is the quality food. SATWIT food, food which is truly pure, of superior quality and of a good balanced diet. It is food that keeps the body healthy. This pure food gives strength, vitality, provides immunity to diseases and illnesses and produces mental, physical and spiritual equilibrium in the whole complex of the human brain and body. This type of foods never produces uric acid and other toxins in the body, it is easily digestive once into the stomach. This is the only food that really protects one's body and mind till very old age and keeps the mind and body in a peaceful and perfect balance.

These are few suggestions of pure food:- Fruit, vegetables, green salads, lentils, milk, curd, cabbage, cheese, fresh butter, hazelnuts, dried fruit, almond, honey, rice and wheat flour.

2. 2nd class is the RAJASIK Food – medium quality food. It is believed that this type of food is a well-balanced diet in our modern way of living. It is a food for vegetarians and partly non-vegetarians. It is a combination of meat, fish, eggs, and with melted butter, sugar, sweets, fried food etc. So these types of food are cooked in oil and grease materials. These foods are being, overcooked, over spiced, and are being served with rich flavour sauces which really diminish the pure substance and value of the food and finally these foods cause all types diseases and pains and acne to the innocent body and mind. The sense of taste is being uncontrolled. These are not healthy to the individual. RAJASIK food is a real hindrance to old age people over fifty and to those who have chosen the spiritual life.

3. 3rd Class is the TAMASIK Food:- This is the lower quality of food. It has a very opposite effect on one's mental and physical equilibrium, and one is easily affected with all sorts of germs and illnesses, because one's immunity system becomes very weak and without resistance. A Tamasik man is someone who lives on stale food, decomposed or dried-up, stale, unclean and rotten food through one's daily life.

Such types of foods, notably fried food, highly sink in grease, butter, margarine, curd etc.. is harmful to the individual body and mind. Fried foods including eggs, meat dishes cooked in grease, cakes made of butter; caseine, or other fatty matters should be consumed in very little quantity by a healthy individual, if possible avoid completely these sorts of dishes for the benefit of one's health.

However, if one knows how to consume pure and high quality food, one would surely improve physically, mentally and spiritually and would definitely stay in good, vigorous and healthy condition and can even live healthily till 100 years.

Clear Proper DIET:
A suitable diet can restore health at any age. The food has a direct effect on the mind as well as the body, but the subtlest part of the food forms the mind.

"By the purity of food one becomes purified in his inner nature; by the purification of his inner nature, he verily gets memory of the self; all ties and attachment are severed." Quote from Chandogay Upanishad.

One should be careful in choosing the foodstuff. Food exerts a tremendous influence over the mind. After a heavy, sumptuous indigestible rich food or meal, it is of great difficulty to get control over the mind. The mind acts like an ape all the time. It runs and wanders and can never be still. The food should be consumed in such a proper way that it can maintain

144

physical efficiency and good health. The good physical and mental of an individual relies much more on a perfect nutrition and a well-balanced diet than on anything else.

In the modern era, the majority of people dig their own graves through their mouth and finally no rest is allowed to the stomach. It is crystal clear that man needs a very little but proper food on this earth to keep life going, but it is a pity to see how they stuff their stomach with all sorts foods, even when they are not hungry and have no appetite, they still stuff their poor stomach. Remember that many diseases have their roots in overloading the stomach.

Be very simple and natural in eating and drinking. "EAT TO LIVE NOT LIVE TO EAT." Evolution is better than revolution. Live a very simple natural life. You should be your own master, not a slave. Have your own menu to suit your constitution. After having a guide, you will be yourself the best judge to select your clear and proper diet.

A well-balanced diet must have four nutrients in the daily life. Whether one is vegetarian or non-vegetarian, four major items must be included in one's major dishes in daily life.

They are salads, fresh vegetables, fresh fruit and raw nuts.

Finally three major aspects are required for a well-balanced diet.

1. One should select nourishing foodstuffs which produce vitality and energy to maintain good health and live a perfect living throughout one's living.
2. One should eat moderately, slightly less than one's hunger, because in this situation the body feels light, active and plenty of energy throughout one's life. Eating as a glutton deforms the body and deteriorates the health system, diminishes efficiency and life becomes short and miserable.
3. The food should be well-chewed and mixed with saliva in the mouth inorder to aid digestion and assimilation. Once the food is in the mouth, it should be chewed thirty to fifty times when taken hard until it is thoroughly insalivated, reduced to a pulp and then into juice, that is turned into liquid. After all, heavy food should be avoided during evening and mainly before going to bed.

However, some few more disciplines: the meals should be eaten slowly, in a peaceful and calm atmosphere. One should keep a very positive mental attitude. One more important fact is that it is of fundamental importance and beneficial for one's health to fast half-day or a day without food once a fortnight or month.

This will help to purify the organs of the body as a whole. While doing this, it is recommended to drink fruit juice, water and especially lemon juice with water. Meanwhile it is a good therapeutic for the benefit of the body. Remember as a car should be always doing its servicing, then it can last longer. Unfortunately we abandon the servicing of our body and mind.

To conclude, a well-balanced diet is a marvelous asset in maintaining the mind in a perfect state of health and equilibrium within a body of perfect and good fitness. If you really want to feel well, eat less. Never hurry when eating, chewing your food properly. Don't eat too great a variety of food at one's meal. Whatever you eat, enjoy it. Let nobody spoil your meal with unpleasant talk and provoking arguments.

A cheerful face, a well decorated dish and table, a beautiful picture or view will help your digestion positively. And last, don't forget that to digest properly, you need a sufficient quantity of oxygen. Don't neglect the deep breathing. Take plenty of fresh air as part of your food.

First advice, don't eat too much food, mainly heavy one, in the evening. You can have heavy meal during the day. Have at least two fruits during the day and plenty of water, at least 5 glasses water, either pure or with lemon during the early morning everyday. If you are at home a whole day, try to drink at least 8 glasses of water throughout the day occasionally.

One most common diet for almost all people of therapeutic yoga is as follows:- One must at least let it be repeated, have two fruits in one daily food intake, salad, leafy vegetables, green vegetables, wheat, bread and pulses and rice mainly red or brown rice, that is unpolished rice is preferable plus raw nuts.

Actually there is no strict rule in yoga that one has to be a complete vegetarian. It all depends upon temperament and climate. Here for a non-vegetarian one can consume fish and liver in certain cases, but meat and chicken should generally be avoided mainly in this modern era as a high use of hormones are used to make these animals become mature before the proper times; there is artificial breeding. About this, people should be very careful and also all canned food must be avoided. But to be a complete vegetarian, this is greatly recommended either from scientific and Yogic point of view.

Here are some basic principles of eating to follow:- (They demand repetition)

1. The fundamental importance is to eat slowly after chewing and crushing the food quite thoroughly. If one is having hard food, the chewing and crushing should be more till the food is masticated to complete liquid in the mouth and well mixed with the saliva.

2. The vital principle is to have dinner, at least two hours prior to going to bed during night. It is not advisable to take tea or coffee before going to bed at night. Don't take more than one or two cups of coffee or tea in a day and if possible try to stop these wholly. If one has a good control and discipline, try to give up the use of tobacco in any form and avoid drinking alcohol.

We all have to die but we have to live in a decent and spiritual way to give examples for the coming generation for a better world.

3. Never consume more food than 85 per cent of the capacity of stomach at any time, that is eaten a little less than one needs.

4. One must avoid drinking water while one is eating. Drink a glass of water half an hour after having eaten food. Take at least five glasses of water as mentioned above and before during 12 hours of the day time.

5. Never consume, if possible, fried, fatty and highly seasoned food. Eliminate if possible hot spices, pickles and sweets. One can prepare one's dishes by using the least amount of spices for flavour.

6. Have food only four times in twenty-four hours, that is have a complete and well-balanced breakfast in the morning, lunch, some light refreshment in the afternoon between 4.00 to 5.00 p.m. and dinner at night. It should be light not heavy food. Finally avoid eating anything in between four fixed hours, but water and juice.

An introduction of diet chart is given as an example to follow:

1. Breakfast, lunch, afternoon refreshment and the dinner is prepared for each yoga practitioner, according to his body condition and nature. But that does not mean that one has to stick to it, but one can follow his or any chart, if it is a balanced diet.

BALANCE AND PROPER DIET:-

Breakfast: 7 to 9 a.m.

1. Tea or coffee drinkers – One cup (if desired) preferable juice or milk.

149

2. Fruit juice, one glass of juice of any type. Example grape or mix-fruit juice.

3. Fresh fruits, one apple or one guava, or one banana or peaches etc..

4. Germinated gram, ¼ cup soaked for a fortnight or more.

5. Wheat bread or toast with butter milk or juice. Cornflakes or oatmeal or wheat germ with milk and sugar (Brown). This is all to one own's 3 habits.

LUNCH AND DINNER – 12 TO 1.00 p.m. and 6.00 p.m. to 8.00 p.m.

1. Mixed salad. Tomato, cucumber, radish, lettuce, carrot etc.. with little salt, pepper and lemon juice or salad dressing, with little olive oil, about a cup.

2. Soup of any kind, one cup.

3. Rice unpolished preferable, bread or brown bread of any kind. (Chapati).

4. Leafy vegetables of any kind.

5. Green vegetables of any kind.

6. Pulses, Mung, mesur, grava, lentil or any kind.

AFTERNOON Refreshment (3.00 p.m. to 5.00 p.m.)

1. Fresh fruit of any kind one or two pieces.

2. Few salted biscuit with tea or milk or juice.

3. Gram or nuts of any type – mix ¼ cup of dry fruits of any type.

This chart becomes meaningful and very important if the following method and principles and requirements are executed sincerely and faithfully.

"Don't forget YOU ARE WHAT YOU EAT & HOW YOU EAT." A very strict advice is given here with real discipline. How to live in the modern era with a healthy body and mind complex.

1. Never eat stale food or veg or anything from the fridge which has been kept longer that 2 days.
2. Never eat just food and snack or any fried food as well.
3. Never eat refined food mainly sugar and rice and etc.
4. Never drink water with food.
5. If possible avoid meat, fish and eggs.
6. Never smoke cigarette or drink alcohol.

By using the above disciplines, your body, mind and soul complex become clean and pure and definitely you can lead a spiritual life.

1. In the morning drink either pure water kept whole night in a copper mug or even lemon water either cold or warm.
2. After lunch, you can have a glass of butter milk or curd.
3. At night, before resting, take a cup of milk either pure or with little raw sugar or honey.

If one follows the above rules, no disease can approach him during his whole daily life.

N.B Common people seem to be very negligent and have no time to drink enough water. They should get used to it at least eight glasses in their daily life.

To get adapted to these above methods of spiritual life, people must get the habit of cultivating the above disciplines and they will have a very controlled mind and senses.

By neglecting the above, people will always have a fragmented mind may be a strong body but the mental attitude and behaviour will be as animalism.

There is no peace and tranquillity of the mind with dual minded.
A trial for at least a month will definitely show its importance. And one must have a will-power, faith with discipline and with regularity in one's daily life.

By following a true living, finally they can build and create pure LOVE within, with sacrifices and acceptance, detachment of mind and discrimination of the mind.

Remember, we all have got a deeper and more fundamental aspect of life with a higher and superior mind, body and soul complex. By using spiritual disciplines, this will take us to our true father, God, the divinity from where we all come from. If not, due to the law of Karma, and the law of reincarnation, we will be retrograded to the ordinary life of animalism and lowest species.

Please help yourself to get out of this circle of birth and death, from these lowest state of lives which are really miserable and low living.

Please try to realize yourself in this transcendent self to become good and to help to produce a world of paradise for the innocent coming generation.

Actually, people don't need to eat a lot as they are doing these days. Discipline is really good health and way to God.

Owing to the wrong way of living, all the 12 organs of the body begin to work upside down. But with disciplines, mainly in spiritual living, all the 12 organs start to function as normally and return to their originality. Once they work properly, one can get all the necessary vital energy "PRANA".

Before I end here, I want to stress the fact that most people are living a fake life by using stale food from fridges and food which has been conserved for days and days and eating too much canned food. Finally, some people get the habit of drinking alcohol. Heart problems and high blood pressures affect them. But what's the use of living that miserable life by using drugs, medicines, stale and tin food. That means you only exist without bliss and never evolve, within the innerself. I prefer not to live life as above mentioned "existing". Better to live a few years with inner realization and become free and liberated by the practice of the Science of Yoga.

1. Study the Name of God
2. A rich man gives name of God to all his children to cheat his innerself.
3. To detach mind from illusion of wife, children, relatives etc, etc..

153

4. A tranquil mind appears on the face. A fragmented mind also appears on the face.

5. As one cannot stay neutral or stable by gain or loss etc.. the same thing happens if the face can appear jovial and happy if the mind is not free and detached and liberated.

There was once a very rich businessman who thought that he could get God just by giving names of deities to all his children.

What happened one day, this man went to attend a lecture where the speaker was giving examples that by taking the names of God before death one can attain liberation. So that rich man thought that he was very clever. So when he came back home, after the speech, he just started to give the names of deities to all his children, because of his idea that one day when he would die, he would call any of his children by names, therefore, he might get mukti, but it is not so easy just to call the name of God once and one could get mukti (liberation), so unfortunately the time of death did come for the rich man to die.

As he was at death's door, all his children were near him and beside him. So to whom he would call, he just told all his children to just look after all the material objects he had accumulated and don't lose any of them, then his body left the soul.

This is an example that God is easy to get if one does the spiritual practices for a very long time. Yoga Japa, Varaigya, Viveka, should be done regularly and sincerely, then one can be liberated.

No control of mind and senses, breathing system and balance diet are being practised by nearly all the modern people nowadays.

CHAPTER 10

SOME PERSONAL SPECIAL SPIRITUAL NOTES

About certain people's behaviour:-

There are people who have everything in life, wife, children, house, car and all luxurious amenities, but still they are mean and miser. Their consciousness is much about their possessions and they always depend on others when others will invite them for meals or dinner or to go out on others' expenses. They make themselves miserable and lead a dog's life. If you really realize, you have to live simply, but don't become a miserly person. If not you will never be happy, even you have every material object.

Live in the world but not of the world. Detach one's mind and discriminate.

Live the spiritual life but not as a pest to others and yourself. Nearly all people on earth think that they have come to change the world with their knowledge. The Ego, hypocrisy, selfishness and avarice predominate. They want to judge and put into practice their own selfish rules, regulations, mainly materially. And they think that they are doing great things in this material world. They are creating troubles and evils and are misled by their own wrong concepts of living. Can they stop growing old and when death is coming, can they stop it and get the instrumental body to become eternal? They have no power of doing this. But why should they want to impose all sorts of material rules and regulations which are really patent by untrue. Most men think of wealth, women and wine; will these them strong and healthy. On the surface only they just show off but inwardly it is just dark and weak.

DHARMA (Righteousness) is to express one's inherent spiritual nature in all actions, internal and external.

Dharma is the flower in the heart of man.
It makes man divine.
It should be the basic ideal of life. It should be the guiding light of life. It should be man's companion in all walks of life.

Unfortunately, it is not like this in this material world, due to the ego and selfish actions. Actually, it is mainly ADHARMA (Unrighteousness) ruling the heart of man in this illusory world. What a pity to see man who is next to God being degraded to animalism all over the world!

Nowadays, man has made immense progress in politics, leadership, business, science, education and knowledge but it is a pity to see no development of themselves within and the precious quality of spiritualism.

It is a pity to see only man evolving in evolution but not in INVOLUTION.

To evolve without involution is the downfall of this precious and next to god species in this Universe. Evolution without INVOLUTION is a disaster to this world, due to the lack of the Science of Yoga and spirituality in human characters and behaviours.

Man must react as from now. It is never too late, there is still time. A bit of my own spiritual experience: "One must experience God. He is everywhere and within everything. It is true that I have been born in my actual family and parents; it is all due to my past Karma. But in my childhood, my parents never taught me how to lead up in this spiritual life. They always lived with their rituals and dogmas and the same routine of following the blind religious system and habits.

Fortunately, I have done my best to do and pursue my own research in this spiritual path. It may be to some of my good, past Karmas that have made me like this and plus my firm belief in the Science of Yoga and meditation, which lands to me in this spiritual life. I have awakened the inner Guru and got an external enlightened Guru to guide me as well in this human form for which I am really grateful. I have pure Love for this spiritual living. But from my experience, it is not that easy, but with sincere and firm determination it becomes possible. My advice to all humans is try to find out the truth and the real path of the spiritual in the human form itself. "Truth will always be victorious." Don't lead an ordinary material life in this illusory world; go back to Godhead as we are of his only image. AWAKEN YOUR INNER GURU. And surely one will get an Enlightened one; this is for sure. Look for the Holy NAME or WORD. Practise the path of Yoga such as Hatha and Astanga Yoga, Meditation, Relaxation, Concentration. Control the mind and senses, get a good spiritual discipline in your life in all actions. Be simple and practical. Have pure love. Everyone has enough time to practise spirituality although involved in this material world. Where there is a will, there is a way. One has enough time to do it, but ignorantly and lazily, one wastes this precious time in only gossiping, concern about others and hankering after only worldly matters. This really sends one backward and retrogrades one from human to lower species.

Have a firm resolution to follow the spiritual life, then one will really see his own life as a paradise and there will be no stress, illness, worries, anger, desires, lust etc, etc, which torment us in life. These are all from our mind and get entangled in the darkness of life and bind us all in the cycle of birth and death, which has been a routine of our daily lives. Please for your own sake, get out of this darkness and awake to divine light with the help of the Ajna Chakra (Third Eye). Get a holy name or word (mantra) from a real enlightened Guru. Explore your innerself which is a reality and true treasure of reality of God. We all live with life-breath (Prana); no one can survive without it. We all, Muslims, Hindus, Christians or from any faith, nationality or ethnic, live due to life-breath. It is everywhere; without it, nothing exists in this universe.
No life breath, no life.
No life breath, no prana.
No prana, no life-breath.

From the mother's womb one gets everything, only no life-breath. Once one is outside the womb, if the baby can't breathe, so no life exists for him. He is already a dead body. Once this life-breath (Prana) gets within, than he is a survived body, when all starts functioning normally.

159

Remember at that stage of a new born baby, its brain is really neutral and pure. So while he starts to grow, it is then that he starts to change due to its environment and upbringing. If the environment is spiritual, it has the great chance to become a great saint, prophet, swami or Avatar etc.

But if his environment is material, he might become very intelligent or literate but a material person and believe and grow in this fake life in which most of our new generations are being grown up. It is a pity to see how they are changing gradually the God created world in to a demoniac one.

Whose is the responsibility and fault? I can say it all depends on the first Guru, that is the mother who is degrading from good to the worst situation.

Long ago, a child lived with the mother till 10 and after that, he was sent to a true Guru. But this has changed as it is difficult to get a true Guru and Gurukool. Now all depends on the work force of the mother, if the mother herself has made no time and has not followed the spiritual path, what is she going to teach the tender child, but only become the slave of the material?

1. A better world can be envisoned; it all depends on the human race. So if one wants to change the world, if one wants to change society, if one wants to change one's family, if one wants a new generation of spirituality to come, first of all one has to change oneself.

Society is made up of individuals; we have to change first the individuals for the better then shall we have a better society.

If for example child is brought up in the environment of worldly people, so what will come of the child is only matter and this child will be copying the environment, behaviour and attitude; this child will get all the bad vibration, bad consciousness and he will never learn spirituality even he turns out to be an intelligent one, this attitude of spirituality will be always missing. That's what is happening in the world of nowadays. Animalism prevails, that's why so many calamities in every field of activity befall us.

2. Actually, no good characters are being shaped by mother or parents.

No good leaders in politics, businesses, science, education are being spirituality brought up. That is the evolution which is being evolved only of objects and material world, where there will be only disgrace and bad influence in society.

When studied properly, animals are found to be better in many cases than humans who have been created as God's image with a better body and mind-complex.

What is happening to the human race of God? They are degraded to animalism because the vibration of Maya, (darkness) is a negative vibration which has pervaded human as a whole. The day of Sodoma and Gomora has already started to filter this beautiful world of God. It is only human who can change himself within else, all humanity in this world will not be saved from horrible and catastrophic situation, if not sooner or later the downfall if this intelligent race will take place. True spirituality transcends all religions.

A child always remains free from tension, worry, fear, stress and is always humble; but if you want to be free from all tensions, worry, fear, stress and be humble you have to follow a child mental attitude or behaviour and become as a child of God and be detached from this world.

When the senses are withdrawn, when the mind is steady and detached and discriminated, when the ego is devoid of its impurities, and merges in the awareness of the self within, one attains eternal bliss and everlasting peace, sat-chit-ananda.

When the mind stops thinking, when the thought waves subside, when the state is neither sleep nor swoon, when one is aware of oneself as pure consciousness, then one realizes the Supreme.

1. Spirituality doesn't mean non-possession of things; it only means non-attachment. A king possessing wealth may be totally unattached while a beggar with torn clothes may be a highly attached man.
2. The greatest worry, anxiety and fear to a man in this world come from himself only and not from any outside source, because the

outside world is all unreal. Once one makes the unreality real, then worry, fear, anxiety, pains, sorrow, loss and gain come to him.

3. One can be amidst living in this jungle, but if one's mind is trained how to detach itself, one is a king of kings in this only world of illusion.

4. Remember that one ounce of practice is better than tons of theory, as it is actually done by nearly 99.999% of people in this material world, because they have become slaves to this only illusory world which is in a constant state of flux.

5. No one can made you happy except yourself.

6. Sickness is in the mind not in the body; one can't be sick until he feels sickness within the mind.

7. It is only the mind that can carry the body where it wants to go, but not the other way around.

8. Once one gets attached as a slave but if one gets detached, he is free and liberated and comes face to face to God, the Almighty.

Now I am again stressing the importance of vegetarianism. Being a vegetarian, I am really living a very peaceful and spiritual life with good sense and humour.

In my youth, when I had to repent, I took action on the spot to change my way of living to that of the spiritual because I was making a big mistake and sin by consuming all kinds of meat. It was only a wrong belief that I was being well fed with the best food of the world, but it was a bad concept. It was only from that time that I made my mind and body systems to tread the true path of spirituality. Before, it was due to the blunder and ignorance of my parents because they have been eating flesh; they think, they are healthy and become strong. It is all a fallacy. According to science, we humans are not meant for eating flesh at all. It has been proved scientifically that we men are vegetarian to eat simple food. But owing to our being unable to control the senses of taste and smell, we overtax our digestive system with carnivore foods which are made for wild animals.

Now I have changed my dietary habit to simplicity and with food that is meant for man. I can prove that my mind and body-complex are really peaceful and with equilibrium.

It is all your mind that can make you weak, strong and tranquil. One can feel strong and free from diseases with less mental problems and bodily problems. Actually people eat flesh and drink alcohol, take all sorts of medicine leading an artificial life ignorantly and not living a natural life.

After stopping to eat such flesh foods, it will take about 10 to 12 years to eliminate all the toxics which have been accumulated in the body organs. By eating such carnivorous food, we are all poisoning ignorantly our body and mind-complex. We get beguiled due to the good taste and flavour. Remember that food with good taste is bad for health. People are fooling themselves and are degrading themselves to animalism.

I have been really fortunate in this human form to have the precious and spiritual opportunity to visit and talk to some of the most inspired and spiritual Gurus of this world. I must say I have been really fortunate and blessed to have and be in their presence and at their lotus feet. I have really been born with a good karma but I don't know in what birth I shall get this spiritual opportunity again. I have been given the grace and chosen to have their darshans and get their spiritual vibrations.

And owing to their grace, I have been able to be very spiritual in this birth. Anyone can start the spiritual Sadhana at any time and at any age and in whatever religion. This can be done. It might a bit hard, but the possibility is within us. Don't act as an escape goat and become a slave of senses and desires.

I can see and feel the Divine light in all human whether bad or good. But it is a pity to see that they can't find it themselves because they get involved too much and submerged themselves in senses of objects in this fake world, which is changeable at every millium of the second.

Secondly, as the mind is submerged in the senses, so there is no break where and when they can get the mind liberated from the strong illusory world (Maya).

It is high time that people learn from a master to withdraw the senses from objects and withdraw the mind from the senses too that they can see that the Divine light is within all of them and I guarantee you that there would be a change in this world with a gift from the spiritual dimension. Remember that although one is sleeping, the Divine light is lighted within, if not he will not see the next day. Look and study the sun; if the sun says that I do not want to give light to the universe even for fraction of a second, what will happen to this beautiful world? All will go to dust again or to nowhere. The Yogi, Sun Air, Water, Earth and Ether never sleep, as they have got the Divine light awakened to keep the Universe going. Only humans born as the only species of the world to have much priority from others, yet, it is painful to see their degradation to backward species. Instead they should try spiritually to return to the Godhead, Almighty Lord. But they let themselves be influenced by materialistic displays, they lose their reality and turn it to unreality. I am quite aware that the material temptation is too strong but fortunately God has given us a formidable brain and body with which we can practise spirituality to attain Him. We can control the mind and senses. We can discriminate and detach ourselves, but unfortunately we ignore the Reality and become the slaves of the unreality.

If man wants to save the world from degradation, he must awake himself to be a spiritual specimen as God himself is.

That is the only path to change everything for the better. It's only by regularity and perseverance, that the Sadhana which has been given by all sages, seers, swamis, prophets, saints and avatara who at any critical time to show us the right path can be accomplished.

The Gita with Lord Krishna as Guru and Arjuna as disciple has given the right spiritual Sadhana for this modern era. Once you practise it with good and sincere intentions, this world becomes a Paradise which comes and flows from within. If the inside is dark, what will happen. You can't see and become blind and start following the blind, as it is said.

However, if you light the divinity within you, then all will be lighted and wisdom of knowledge starts to bloom from within yourself; this is for sure. The individual practice of Yoga is a great need in our daily life. Don't waste your precious and spiritual time and get muddled and entangled in the material world. Use it simply to advance yourself towards God. This is possible. When one is able to overcome worldly pleasures and pains, attractions and repulsion, one doesn't experience simply a blank and void but one experiences a spiritual awakening. The ignorant let live the stupid or fool. "Ignorant fais vivre L'imbecile et fais aussi vivre le stupide," goes a French saying.
The stupid or fool let live the ignorant.

Some spiritual instructions are:-

1. Practise Pranayama, withdraw the senses from the external objects. Discriminate the Real from the unreal. Detach the mind as from the unreal to Reality. Meditate on the Atman, the eternal into Nirvikalpa. Samadhi. Realize your oneness with the Supreme.

2. Withdraw the senses from the objects and withdraw the mind from the senses. Establish yourself in your inner self centre or Atman.

3. Pure love and faith and reason should walk hand in hand to herald the birth of wisdom.

4. The essences of Gita are the main spiritual core in human life. And these are meant only for human to practise them spiritually with love and faith.

In the Gita. KRISHNA is the Guru (God) who guides the Disciple – Arjuna in the battle field of life:

1. He is the Guru- Arjuna the disciple.
2. He teaches Arjuna the Science of Yoga.
3. He teaches him to do only good actions in whatever situation. Do good action to kill the bad ones.
4. With every breath remember "Me" in whatever situation. Remember the Guru (God) name, with Para, Love and feel Him within one self.

This is the reality of the human life in this illusory world. God is the eternal and spiritual and the rest is all illusion.

1. Self-realization is not achievement or attachment. It is the discovery of the self in one's own heart. Just like milk poured in milk, oil in oil and water in water, when mixed become one even so the knower of the self becomes one with the supreme Brahman, the known.
2. He is established in wisdom who is ever undisturbed, who is actionless, who is extremely solemn and deep like the ocean.

3. Bliss is something to be achieved. It is there always, but obscured. Remove the veil of ignorance and Reality the immortal Bliss will be there.
4. The ignorant longs for results and engages in action with the idea of doership and enjoyership.
5. There is no ignorance outside the mind. The mind alone is Avidya, the cause of bondage, of transmigration; when that mind is destroyed all else is destroyed.
6. All beings are by nature pure consciousness. It is due to ignorance that they appear to be different from it.

If you don't want to realize yourself to be one with God, others are the same as Karma varies from one to the other. But at least for health's sake, try at least to practise Asanas and Pranayama to escape from these mental torturing, noxious and modern diseases which are spreading and contaminating the human body and mind.

Now, many old people talk about freedom and liberty. How can they have these when they themselves are involved in the material world and a slave to it? And what surprising is that they are still money-minded and never be satisfied with themselves.

The father, grand-father or grand-grand-father instead of shirking their responsibilities, should live with their little or grand-children and be with them, share their childhood and bring them up with love and do sacrifice for them. The old really fear being rejected. They are not free and have liberty, of which they are talking, they are running away from themselves.

I am not flattering or boasting anyone but this fact is real. I have my own soul-mate who has done all his 4 ashrams. Now he is living blissfully with his little children. He appears really human and spiritual at the age of 70 still looking after his mother who is bed-ridden since very long and his ailing wife. That is what is called real love and sacrifice, freedom and liberty. He knows Himself and he sees this self in all, either young or old. Pray God be always with him till death do part him. He is one to be born in a very high spiritual family in next birth. I am sure for this.

What comes out of Pure love.
Out of Pure love comes Pure love.
Out of Jealousy comes Jealousy.
Out of Spiritual comes the Spiritual.
Out of the Ego comes the Ego.
Out of Hatred comes Hatred.
Out of Worry comes Worry.
Out of Fragmented mind comes Fragmented mind.
Out of Yogi comes Yogi.
Out of Sacrifice comes Sacrifice.
Out of Seed comes Tree.
Out of Tree come the Seeds.
So out of good and Pure mind in human come children with good and pure mind in this world, then this world can be saved from these five often

scoundrels in the world. The five are often politicians, businessmen, scientists, educationists and parents, people responsible for the coming generation. There is a speed without, but a slow evolution within. Remember when one goes too fast, what happens? He often stumbles and falls down and the consequences are disastrous. I am not generalizing about the five mentioned above; there have been some good individuals among them, but very few.

Now PURE LOVE; Nowadays it is a pity to see how people, mostly materialistic bent, have doubt about this purity of love and are going against it because their mind is impure, attracted to unreal objects of worldly matter, and it becomes fragmented, so how can they appreciate or have real love and know what Pure Love. It is all a matter of being brought up in this field of spirituality from very young.

1. Love and sacrifice are two pillars of this world. Remember that it is with love, that one is born.
2. Remember that with love that the five elements keep on going, if there is disharmony, the five elements will split apart and disaster will befall the universe.
3. Without love, God wouldn't have created our beautiful world with humans as the highest species. It's deplorable, however, to see how human beings have polluted the world by a shortage of pure love. We find rather selfish and ignorant motives.

And by listening and following Him, I really get stuck to my Guru. I can say that I really know who I am, where I come from, where I am going and what I must do to follow the real path. But I always beg Him, God, the Almighty, to let me have the chance to come again in this human form to fulfil my spiritual life, so that I can break the barrier of the circle of birth and death. But whatever I am feeling, this is due to the blessing of my Guru. I hope I would be able to come out from. I have been given this net of birth and death in this human form. I have been given the name "Surendrhananda". which is a spiritual name (initiation) referred in the Gita "Surendralokam."

" Chp II, vase 19-20.

1. Try first to control the mind
2. Control the Senses
3. Discriminate
4. Detachment
5. Have Pure Love and sacrifice
6. Practise the Reality, that is the Yoga path
7. Always live with Satsanga, where the Master guides you.

Among all the species in this world, Human is said to be the most intelligent, but to my experience, Human is the most stupid, silly and ignorant with a weak brain, because people want to conquer this material world by hook or by crook. Eventually, they end up by destroying themselves and the beautiful nature around, making this world a hell to live in. Scientists, politicians, businessmen, educationists and finally the material behaviour of mothers are causing this deteriorating havoc to this world; again, I am not generalizing.

Even animals have a sort of discipline in their daily lives, but human beings despite the great fantastic Law of Reality and discipline, bypass them and lead a completely material life without any control. What they call progress is simply but I call digressing and transgressing of their own self. They use evolution to very extreme for material objects. Instead they should involve themselves with the innerself, with the help of the Spiritual life by using the natural discipline of Yoga and stick to the Law of Reality and nature. These are gifts given by God.

Remember this universe is infinite and we must all go for the real soul which exists in all, either animate or inanimate. I have always said I am a Universal man. I do not belong to such a community or country, village, town or to any caste, creed, religion or colour. I am born the same as others. I believe only in the race of Mankind, with others as my brothers and sisters. By spiritual extentions, one can come out free from this suffering world because once one is born, one must, as a human species, join the infinite, not to come back in to the net of the circle or birth and death.. One has to transform oneself and the innerself Spiritually and to lead a simple and non-attached life from this world of objects.

The most miserable people in this world are those who really rely and trust the material objects of this world, mainly those who rely on first money, wealth and women. They think that they are making name and fame and that they are happy, but really they are making fools of themselves. All these materials are fake and generate troubles, stress; the two real enemies in our lives are the uncontrolled mind and senses. People really let their mind and senses become their master. Once they get stuck in these, they go from worst to worst and that is the downfall of humans. The world is becoming a furnace for humans to live in, with all sorts of devastating calamities, still to befall us in the near future.

It is high time that humans turn to the Reality by a waking up of their innerself. On the contrary, they are forgetting their trueself and becoming ignorant, indifferent, hypocrite, selfish and finally darkness is invading them. The Divine light is within all of us, but being engulfed in this illusiory world, they are lost as the "Brebis egarée" the lost lamb in the dense forest, which is this material world.

S = Spirit

O = Omniscient, Omnipresent, Omnipotent

U = Universe = Infinite, like the blue sky, Akasha

L = Love, purity of love such as a little child loves the mother.

Prana

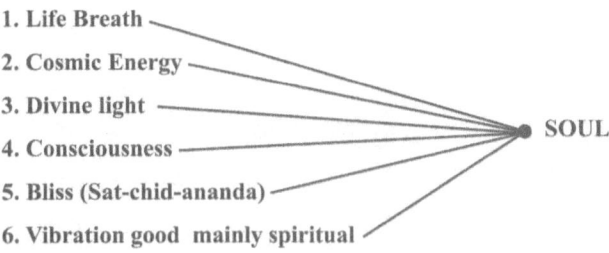

1. Life Breath
2. Cosmic Energy
3. Divine light
4. Consciousness
5. Bliss (Sat-chid-ananda)
6. Vibration good mainly spiritual

SOUL

Practise these above mentioned; one will get transformed into transcendental as one with Almighty God.

The SOUL can be realized only by following the Scientific path of yoga. Yoga is of prime importance in one's daily life; without this practice of Yoga, the individual life becomes shattered with nervous breakdown and one becomes slave to this illusory and material life and can't communicate to his innerself and become an ordinary individual and never come out of this circle of birth and death. Finally, one can never have permanent inner happiness which is Sat-chit-ananda "BLISS" in one's daily life. Life becomes always miserable and full of mental and bodily stress till death.

Actually men can be generally classified under four categories in this world. According to me, I consider man as two races.

1. Male and female from whom procrastination can exist and that has made this population in the world.

However, the four categories are:

1. Ordinary or common men of this world, 99% of which I can say are wholly material.

2. Then come the Siddhas, they struggle spiritually by Yoga path and with their good actions of past and present can realize their perfect nature afterwards and who are distinguished from an incarnation by this struggle.

3. The Nitya Siddhas who accompany the incarnation just as fragrance always be side by side of the flowers, or such as rays always related to the sun.

4. The incarnation one who is always independent. He is already the truth. He is born as illumination within. He seems to struggle for realization, but only intended to teach men how to follow the path to liberation. He comes with good spiritual examples to guide his erring children how to behave in such as to get away from illusory and material life.

Practise rigorous discipline to purify and steady the mind and to fix it on Atman or the Supreme Self. This is the highest austerity.

"You are what you eat"

This sentence is well-said, but people misunderstand it. It is meant if someone eats a well-balanced food or diet, he will be a well-balanced man. That means he is getting all the necessary, carbohydrates, protein, fat, minerals and vitamins in his body and indeed all the 12 organs are working properly, then he is a well-being man and his spiritual life will take him to the Almighty kingdom of God. This is for definite, I must say it.

So it is sad to see that people cannot control their senses and they develop the bad habit of eating meat, eggs, fish, as the Europeans have done and Asiatics too have developed the bad habit of eating spices, chillies, curry etc, etc, in excess.

After all, we humans have not been born to eat meat etc., because scientifically it has been proved that these carnivorous foods have not been made for humans as per their stomach, intestines, mouth, teeth and saliva which are not meant for these above foods. But it is a pity to see people, in order to gratify their senses, have gone out of their control and are damaging the law of nature and Divinity. It is said, the world will evolve, I agree, but to what situation, devilishly or spiritually? The trend indicates that the demonical world is developing in the near future; no one will be able to repair the damage done. * I have done research and proved that even the heavy-weight lifter, if he is a vegetarian, he is better than the one who is a meat-eater. The problem is a balanced diet. People don't want to understand that is why all the governments have to invest huge sums of money in medicines and hospitals. This is a waste of money.

Nowadays, people seek matter first and spirit afterwards, even if they are aware of this. Instead people should reverse this process. The heart also must be free from any vile and selfish motives. Most People love God for personal benefits, thus they really love the world but not God, That's why people can never be true, devotees. The true devotee loves God just for the joy of loving Him because God is their Beloved.

There is fasting which is recommended by the Guru to the disciple only on spiritual basis. I can accept one day fasting which is good for health, still the body should be supplied with soft or liquid food. A car without petrol, oil, or water and electricity can't run. This you must accept surely.

Consider these points:

1. Wrong way of eating without discipline daily.
2. Wrong food, and control of the senses, mouth and tongue taste.
3. Wrong way of sleeping, not enough time to sleep.
4. Wrong way of doing exercises, either too much and the wrong time or not enough and still at wrong time.
5. Wrong way of behaving in works with family or friends or in society. Become selfish with ego, hypocrite, big liar to enjoy themselves. No one can trust no one etc...
6. Acting wrongly. The actions are wrong to each other. Remember that all actions good or bad have its reaction. KRISHNA is the example in Gita.

1. In this world of today, even some Gurus are becoming impostors as this material world is too alluring with negative vibrations. People should beware of many AGURUS, who come even for their own selfish means, so that they can live their material in their own way.

2. For God's sake don't misuse spirituality in the name of religion for selfish ends. If this happens, their will be no truthful being in this world, and no one would be able to trust anyone in whatever field of activity. And eventually, this world will end as the well-known cities of Sodome and Gomor as mentioned in the Bible; these cities were destroyed after having gone against the law of nature and divinity.

This will be a very sad end. Hope this won't happen if humans start to realize his innerself, that his happiness dwells within with the conquest of the ego.

Actually five categories of human beings are mainly responsible for the degradation of this beautiful world created by God. I accept that there must be evolution, but without involution these scoundrels are making this terrestrial paradise into a furnace of Hell. They are and this has to be repeated again I don't generalize:

1. Politicians
2. Businessmen
3. Scientists
4. Educationists And
5. The role played by the first Guru "Mother" who is irresponsible and too much involved in objects and material living. The parents, Mother and Dad have let themselves been seduced to the evolutionary material world. It is all their faults if the new generation is becoming out of control and fully materialistic.

179

There is no more Divine Mother now, those only materialist, mothers who are running after this fake evolution material and illusory world. So it is sad to say that they are the irresponsible mothers who are the production of all these materialistic Politician, Businessman, Scientists and Educationists.

Owing to material way of upbringing the innocent children in this illusory world by the materialist mothers, (not all) people are brought up without involution and without any spiritual discipline. So this causes the degradation of the beautiful world made by the Almighty. What a pity and sadness. Mothers and women, it is time for you all to wake up and take your responsibility so that the world can be out of this deplorable situation.

Actually, there are many people in this material world with wrong ideas because they think they can get bliss by staying in ignorance. They are completely wrong as they will never get bliss in the way they are thinking. On the contrary, they are spoiling the infinite word of 'bliss' into a wrong theory of showing off.

But as I have already said before, the ignorant let live the stupid or fool and the stupid or fool let live the ignorant.

When can this kind of above characters realize bliss, a secret spiritual path? Sat-Chid- Ananda can be obtained only by spiritual practice (Sadhana) to realize the innerself. By staying ignorant, people automatically become hypocrites, selfish and full of the devilish ego.

180

It is all pretention to con or cajole people, to show off good character on the surface and make people believe just to show off, but inside many people in the dark; even darkness is better than these characters.

Tantric Tradition

Tantra is also a collective little part of yoga that covers a vast range of practical teaching leading to the expansion of human consciousness and the liberation of primal energy (Kundalini). The unifying principle behind the diverse systems of tantra is that the material world and its experiences can be utilized to attain enlightenment.

Today, some schools of thought and people describe tantra as sexual practices promising longer ecstasy and better orgasms, increased stamina. But this is a superficial interpretation of the Tantric Tradition. The real tantra aims to awaken "kundalini", the dormant potential force in human personality.

Although there are many branches of Tantra, the practices common to all systems leading to transcendental awakening are mantras (vibrational tuning through sounds), yantras concentration symbols to liberate the consciousness, charkas realization of psychic centers, mandalas perception of macrocosmos in microcosmos, tapasya, practices of self purification, Raja Yoga integral yoga. Pranayama yogic breathing practices, self surrender, shaktipat, transmission of energy and frantic initiations, a process incorporating all of the above imparted by a qualified master to a deserving disciple.

Tantra advocates a pattern of life which integrates the faculties of the intellect and the heart. The functions of the intellect are discrimination and concentration and those of the heart are seeing the unseen, having a glimpse of the transcendental or cosmic consciousness beyond the material.

He who believes in the illusion of plurality moves on the wheel of birth and death. The dualist is never free from fear. He is miserable. Bondage lies in the belief "I am the body." Liberation lies in constant faith. I am Light, Self, Brahman, that is always meditate, "I AM BRAHMAN" by melting the ego with the Absolute. One who indentifies himself with the body has fear from all sides. Renounce the idea that the body is the self and identify it with the fearless, immortal Brahman. You will become absolutely fearless.

Bliss is not something to be achieved. It is always there, but obscured; remove the veil of darkness and ignorance and realize the immortal Bliss.

Worry and creasing in the mind constitute a living death.

To become divine is the aim of life. Do not leave the world empty-handed. Amass the supreme wealth of Atman. Do not miss the golden opportunity this life gives you for God realization . Study the sacred books, the book of

182

life, again and again. The opening words of a book are "You are all pervading son." Live in the Eternal. Tat twam Asi. Thou art that." Realize this and be free and divine as God is; we are all here to do this, but people get themselves entangled in this object and material world of slave and attachment and get themselves in the net of birth and death.

The dualist is never free from fear. He is miserable.

Liberation and freedom do not lie in this illusionary and material living. They are all within the "Self" because people believe in false and illusionary objects to be real and they forget the SELF in this unawakened world of unreality.

1. Without a spiritual master, there is no knowledge of wisdom. Without the knowledge of wisdom, there is no God. Without realizing God, no one knows He Himself or His innerself and who is He.
2. He who is not affected in the least when he is injured by others and who is worshipped by nobody is a wise man.
3. I wish that there are no names for God as He is unlimited and infinite. But it is a pity to see the pseudo religious people give names to God in each religion and turn him to be limited and finite. Instead I prefer people practising Yoga of Love and see Him within themselves; then they can reach the infinite and see Him in everything, animate and inanimate. Of course, practice is not only theoretical

(My spiritual relation with Baba is a part of my Past Karma).

1. He himself advised me in a darshan, to follow my Guru as there is nothing higher than a Guru. He is the gateway to God-hood in human life.

2. As I am a lover of KRISHNA and his Yoga teaching, I have this always in mind because people always say Sai Ram but in my mind I always ask Baba taken in a Godman on earth. Please reveal to me if your are Saikrishna, and surprisingly 3 or 4 years ago, a relative from Australia sent me a nice photo of Baba taking in a ceremony and in that picture, when developed it appeared as Krishna himself. So there are mysteries in our spiritual life and can't be explained as it is beyond explanation. It is all the real faith within oneself, either one believes it or not. But these mysteries are all truth.

1. In the epic of Ramayana, Rawan was the demon and always against his brother Bibishan who was a faithful servant to the reality of God. Finally as a little brother, he was kicked out from the building of demon by Rawana, his elder brother.

2. In the life of Sai Baba, he is either a Godman or a Mangod, whatever you believe. He also suffered the same fate, his elder brother was against his spiritual mission in his life and I don't feel any surprise when I am a lover of God and have faith in reality by being thrown out by my nearest relatives who are a materialist, but I do always respect and forgive them because they are born like this

184

due to their bad past Karma. These materialists make us, spiritual people, more and more powerful in our spiritual mission in this human form.

Humans should remain Daivic, pure with love, not asuric demonic, selfish ignorant, sensual and hypocrite.

Krishna in the Geeta teaches us the three main spiritual path which were taught to Arjuna as a fervent devotee to Krishna. They are:

1. To practise Yoga as a Science throughout one's whole life. Make it part and parcel of living.
2. To awaken the sleeping Guru who lies within all of us. Then you get the outside one to lead you, and
3. Must do good actions disinterestedly. Actions should be done Pure with sacrifice and Love. Every action, good and bad, has its reaction throughout one's life. Do you work as duty.

After realization has been acquired by practising the above mentioned, then you will come to inspire and have experience of God and get to experience three main spiritual sources in daily life. They are:-

1. The PRANA – LIFE Energy and Vital or Cosmic Energy, without it, nothing can survive.
2. The Divine light which can be disclosed as the Third Eye (Ajna Chakra). Without Divine light, one always lives in darkness. It is always there, but not realized because the material illusionary world is too strong in daily life. Instead of becoming a servant to

185

the Divine light, people become servants to fake and illusory material world and fall in the circle of birth and death ignorantly.

3. Without Air breathing in and out, can someone survive? No. It is a two way traffic. Inhaling or exhaling, both must be there and one cannot stay without breathing. That is the "Word" which God blows in the nose to get it. That's what we call PRANA. Air is what the scientists can't define or can't go through. No one can disapprove this indefinable Energy. In another word, we can say VIBRATION. Nothing stays without Vibration, everything vibrates. No vibration, no life.

All these have been realized by Sages, Prophets, Swamis, Avatars, Seers and so on. However, every one has to realize it internally. That's why we say that practical spiritual knowledge should be carried on by all humans to reach the highest goal, one with God as we are all in his image. You believe it or not, that is the reality in human life.

When most of the materialist people in the world with their lowest level of mind see or come into contact with a spiritual man, either they think this spiritual man mad or stupid or fool because of his being unattached to worldly material objects or blame him that He is missing a lot in his life by not enjoying wealth, women and wine and other materialist pleasures. I can say on the contrary that the genuine spiritual man is the happiest man in this world as he has been able to detach his mind and senses by not living in the furnace world of illusion. He has become a pure and strong mind where nothing unreal attracts him and while living and working among the fools, he never gets contaminated by their evil behaviour and conduct in this mayavic world.

The real fools are those people who are entangled in the unreal world and they are pretending that this unreal is real as they labour under a delusion. They are not free from any adversity. They are weak and living like an oak tree, four hundred or more but of no use. They live in Rajasick and tamasick life and can't get away form this bondage either in foods, lifestyle ways of thinking, in gossip and frustration very restlessness and disillusionment. Such is their lot till their death do part them.

In my experience and inspiration, people need very little to live happily and harmoniously in this world. We create our own problems and failures but blame others or sometimes the an innocent "God", we always seek for scapegoats and rationalize.

"Never judge others or criticize others, when we do this, we are doing harm to our own self, because we are all one and one in all; due to ignorance, hypocrisy, people don't come to realize this, goes a saying"

We are never alone. God is always with us. We become blind due to our slavery to this unreal world. We are all of the five elements, water, air, fire, earth and ether (Sky infinite). While doing concentration, one can find it by seeing the colours with the Ajna Chakra, (eye brow) Third Eye. Water is white colour, Air is green, fire is red, earth is yellow and ether (Akasa) is blue, the infinite. This is an example to show how we are all the same, but we get entangled in name, fame, status, wealth and people make themselves divided in groups or ranks or classes and build up a complex of superiority among themselves. After all, we all are born from women and have parents and we all will die in the same way, that is the body will be disintegrated.

We all have to come and go; this is the law of nature. Nowadays, people are forgetting nature and going in modernism and the Information Technology era against nature and destroying the welfare of God state. We are turning this world into Sodome and gomore. We people of this world have to be blamed. We are straying from the real track. Like a train going out of rail, we are witnesses to a deplorable state of affairs. It is not that, we are one with Him?

What is meditation and how to attain it? First it should start practically with the process of Yoga and to follow the eight path or fold of Astanga Yoga. Why? Because you have been of the world process since your childhood. As it is said, you have to be in the world, but not of the world.

So the only way to come out of this is to practise the above mentioned Yoga path and then finally when your body mind and soul complex has been synchronized, then it is really possible to do Meditation, which is a 24- hour process of reminding God through your only breathing system of inhaling and exhaling. Once you reach this plane, then you are sure to, have attained the goal of meditation, Superconsciousness is one with Him God, the Almighty and what human has come on this earth to do is to breakout from the circle of birth and death. As you are born, you must suffer. That is the Law of nature. No one can escape this law once he is born.

So one has to practise spirituality fervently, to get to meditation for 24 hours. It is only in this human life that it is possible to do it and the only way to get out from this net. Don't become a slave to materialism. On the contrary, one must become his own Master by finding a True and real Master, who can also help one to get out of this material junk of misery and suffering.

When there is happiness, sorrow is also there, so one must practise the middle or neutral way, the only gateway of humanity.

Till now if I have witnessed and seen mysteries and miracles, it is all due to opportunity and spiritual luck.

1. Once, my soul-mate had his wife in a coma after she had got a brain (tumor) vein broken and her case was serious. I remember he called me first and I rushed immediately to the Clinic. When I reached there, I went to see her with very positive one-pointed mind, that God must give her life again and if she could still have the chance to live again. I could vision that the divine light still in her was very positive, and soon I heard my friend calling me to say that his wife was out of danger. I call this a mystery and God listens to you when you have pure love and pure mind while worshipping Him. He is with us all.

2. One nephew of mine from my sister's side had a serious accident, a very young boy and he went into the coma for a few days. And the doctor condemned him also, that he would be no more. So I went to see him in the hospital with a very positive one pointedness mind and with great determination and I asked Almighty God to give him a chance to come again and surprisingly I could see the Divine light within him. The parents were staying with us for some period while he was in the hospital and after few days, the doctor called his parents and said that this was incredible: he was saved from danger and they would meet him again. These are what I call miracles and mysteries of the human mind.

3. There is the case of another nephew from my brother's side. He and his sister had lived together with me since early childhood and now they are in England, far from me. But a few years ago, they phoned me to inform about the serious illness of my nephew; he could not move and had to stay in bed at the hospital. Although I was far from him. I became very positive with one-pointed mind and asked my own self for his cure and later he came out of his dangerous situation. These are all His (chamakar), mysteries and miracles, either one believes it or not. These are true revelation in my spiritual life till now

Mother role

In the material world, the real ashram (Hermitage) is the house where the first and real Guru who gives birth to children is the mother, but it is very painful to say that in this world and house, the mother is not doing her work as it should be done. She has lost the tract and believes that this material world is real and like the 'Brebis égarée' the lost lamb, she goes astray. The mothers themselves are not grown up with this treasure of spirituality, so how can they pass it to the new generations? Mothers should change and take their responsibility as spiritual mothers. If not, it will be too late when this world will go to a degradation level, when and where it will be impossible to remedy it. It will become a real Hell to my knowledge. The world itself can be a Paradise or Hell depending on the character or behaviour and mental attitude of the people themselves. Now as I have said the house is an ashram, definitely the body is the temple of God where God resides. It is up to mothers to bring up their children in the spiritual way along good and not bad direction.

Homes should be filled with a kind and generous father with a true and loving mother. When they are thus filled, animated, by spiritual dimension, the world will be better civilized, intelligence will rock the cradle, justice will prevail, wisdom will reign in the legislative hall and above all, the door of heaven will pour the sweet spirit of liberty.

The following precepts have to be cultivated from the tender ages:
1. I am the Reality. I am in Reality and the Reality is within me.
2. I am the light, I am in the light and the light is within me.
3. I am the love, I am in the love and the love is within me.
4. I am the breath, I am in the breath and the breath is within me.
5. I am purity, I am the purity and purity is within me.

6.   I am the spirit soul, I am in the spiritual soul and the spirit soul is within me.

7.   I am consciousness, my subconscious is clean and pure and I am in the superconciousness.

People should know how to adjust, accommodate and practice these principles in their lives, then all else becomes easy and life itself is sweet.

Bliss makes one become spiritual, spiritual makes one become bliss.
Divinity turns one naturally up to God.
Devil turns one artificially down to animalism.

Materialist people of the world with the luxurious and comfortable possessions such as houses, cars, wives, children, money etc.. think that they have got bliss and happiness. Yet they get happiness only in the external which is temporary. At any time, the dark atmosphere of distress may overcome and surround them. By living ignorantly, they think that they have bliss. It can't be true; it is just in words and a misconception of Bliss.

Only a spiritual living can lead to Bliss: the one who has sacrificed by practising all sorts of Sadhana, or spiritual disciplines in his life. It is not that one accumulates a fortune and by living in extravagance. Lead a simple life. Simplicity is divinity when one can discriminate and detach one's mind and live with the pure love within and see equality in everyone. He can see Himself in all and all within Him.

Ignorance, stupidity, foolishness, greed, miserliness, money, wealth, wine, women etc, etc.. make people blind and believe that this illusionary world is real due to their blindness. They just see the objects, but never practise to see the subject within. God underlies all the material world and objects. With spiritual practice, one can see behind all those delusive objects and will come to know His plays behind all things.

"A wise man having understood that the body, senses, mind, intellect are entirely distinct from imperishable Brahman roams about happily, goes a saying."

Divine life or Yoga does not ask man change his religion or run away from home or life and live in solitude as a miserable man who is running away from all his responsibilities like a coward. What is needed is to detach the mind from the objects of the world and attach it to the Lord for twenty four hours regularly, which is called 24 hour meditation.

Though the body is full of filth and disease, one can taste the Divine Essence in the body alone. It is the abode or temple of the Lord. Therefore, keep it strong, clean and healthy by all means Ref: to my book, <u>Human body in the real temple of God.</u>

To be selfish is to be indifferent, ignorant and hypocrite, which are demoniac life. To perceive diversity is demonical life, to see unity is divine. To identify oneself with the body is demonical, but to identity

193

oneself with Atman, Brahma is divine life. Divine life leads one to immortality, but evil life drags one from death to death and cannot escape the cycle of birth and death.

Most people are nourishing their body with an ill-balanced diet everyday. They have become too much. 1. Tamasic 2. Rajasic

It is very few that are nourishing their soul with the Satwick food, that is a balanced diet or even to go beyond the Satwick food.

In my books, you will find a chart on a balanced food and how to eat daily. This is only a spiritual advice. It is up to you to follow them or you can make your own balanced food daily.

The more we are involved in wordly pleasures and enjoyments, the more do we get bound and entangled and the more difficult it becomes for us to be free from bondage.

Human beings are becoming worse than animals in their way of eating all kinds of food to please their senses and the tastes from childhood. Even a dog is fasting within a fortnight. But humans are losing all their spiritual values dormant within. What a denigrated race for one who is born with great opportunity to return to God kingdom!

One who has misused the human form and does not become self-realized is no better than a dog.

Wherever you go, you can witness the depravity of humans. They gather in groups in functions, follow blindly dogmas and ceremonies or enjoy themselves with relatives and friends. Most of the talking is about material world or gossip about relatives and friends or about their country politics or as it is actually about the diseases and illnesses afflicting people of all ages. That is disgusting as they come to forget their own self. Instead they should gather to talk about good things such as love and spirituality, instead of wasting their times absurdly and become either mentally or physically weak.

A child always remains tension free. Similarly adults can also be tension free if they consider themselves as the children of God.

If you could control the speech, the mind, the breath and the senses, you will think by a pure mind and control the self by the Self. Then this is for sure that you will no more return to this illusionary world.

Theft, injury to others, falsehood, hypocrisy, lust, anger, pride, haughtiness, discord, enmity, dishonesty, envy, overindulgence in sexual matters or any objects, wine and gambling. These fifteen evils beset men and have indeed their source in wealth. Therefore, one who is desirous of obtaining the highest good should brush aside evil known as wealth.

The deceptive characters think this is my body and they go astray. They mistake the body a mere creation of mind to be their own and themselves.

They are deluded by the false notion of "I" "Me" and "Mine". They think "He is different" and thus wander in the unlimited wilderness of ignorance.

We always think that by changing this or that condition, we will be in a more comfortable position in this world. But in the new conditions also, we find ourselves surrounded by new problems; this is a vicious circle. Unless we realize that the source of happiness is within us, we may live anywhere and in whatever conditions and remain stressed and miserable.

The real Ashram (house of spirituality) is one's home and the body is the real temple of God. But if people are full of the Ego, hatred, lust, envy, jealousy, ignorance, hypocrisy, selfishness etc.. and always waste their time in gossiping and talking bad and criticising others; what kind of house it will be? It will be only a real hell in this world itself.

Nowadays, in almost every home, you can only hear and see people deeply involved in worldly news and events. You hardly hear any prayers or word of God and thinking or talking about the Lord.

People think of God for a while often going to pray for a show and then completely forget God and their Innerself.

Nowadays, the greatest sin in conjugal life (sacred wedding) is that when the bride and bridegroom get married, they vow before God fidelity to each other. But in many cases, divorce ensues soon as they can't go on for several material reasons and personal conflicts due to characters and

196

behavioursAdultery is rampant. Instead of living a peaceful and harmonious life, bringing up their children along the spiritual path in order to keep this Law of wedding very firmly till their ends, they really live or lead a very miserable and distressful life. How can they be happy? They just show people that they are happy superficially only, but interiorly, they are filled with mental disorders and are mostly neurotics; we, therefore, witness broken families living only with stress, disharmony and chaos. That's the way this world is being built up in a negative way. At least, these couples should learn and practise karma yog or Sanyasa Guru such as Swaraswatti of Bihar School of Yoga. His book is really a limelight to conjugal life and how to lead a happy living and how to bring up the children as well.

In this day and age, there is a material revolution, but not a spiritual evolution.

Instead of spiritual evolution, man has gone too far against the will of God and his ownself and plunged deeply in the revolution of a material world. This will bring about a great deterioration to our paradise world in the coming future. So humans have to bring great reforms in their lives, what I mean is a spiritual reform from childhood. Our parents have not learnt and practised the same and they have brought up their children only in a revolutionary world of materialism. So to come out of this furnace, the children must practise the spiritual evolution and get transformed in an evolution of character. From childhood, they should practise the quest of the innerself by following the great path of yoga, which was introduced by the great seers of ancient India from time immemorial, mainly the Sage

197

Patanjali, Yoga Sutra which is meant for common and ordinary people of this age.

Religions have been established by the prophets, sages and saints. They came at the ripe moment, when they were needed to reform people who have gone out of the track of Reality. At that crucial time, prophets, sages and saints were of great help in the areas among the people who needed them.

But the greatest aberration is to see how their followers have often misunderstood them and mis-followed them, distorting their teachings and eventually baffling other followers in the wrong way. Really to say, all religions lead only to one goal, that is towards Divinity. A religions person is one that follows spirituality and the right path throughout his life. This is the art of living in life.

However, there are the Sufis (the mystics in Islam) as good examples to people. They are really not so bigoted and their way and practice in their daily living is peace and love of God. Now you have the Hindu itself or the, Sanatanan Dharma. First of all "Hin" means stay away from "du" such means violence. So in everyday life, one must live away completely from the violent way of living, that is living a life of non-violence even (ahimsa), the killing of even animals. The Hindu evinces such practice "Sanatana" means eternal and "Dharma" means the right duty in every day life of a person. So one should do his eternal right duty with good actions in daily life whatever the circumstances. He holds the belief that God will protect him against wrong-doers. When one lives it as it should be, then one will experience the same. To live the Sanatanan Dharmas, one should not harbour the worst enemy within, that is the Ego and fear. Fear and the ego are the hardcore of our everyday life in this material world.

Right living is to go within the innerself, to know oneself by practising the path of the Science of Yoga, which is not a religion but a Science and an art of living. After all, we are all of the five elements: earth, fire, wind, water and ether. We are all children of God who has created us. We are all born in only one way; we all come out from the wombs of the mother, that is the Big Bang in my own inspiration and experience spiritually. So it is crystal clear that all of us are born from our past actions and duty and we come to such and such parents due to our own chosen past actions and duty from our past birth. Once we are born as the human species, we have to try hard to lead a right living, even if we have not been guided from our parents inorder to break our circle of birth and death. It is the good actions and right duty of our past together with our good actions and right duty in this birth that can eliminate the crucial net of birth and death.

It is high time that people realize it and then the world will be really a terrestrial paradise for each one to live peacefully.

I have witnessed in my daily living how much time people are wasting in unnecessary objectives and material talking, gossiping and involving in what does not concern them. Instead they should try to find out the real path and duty and to meditate on God in their daily life. It is all a waste of human life by indulging in wrong and bad ways of living which bring people back to the animal life in their next birth.

I know that the material life is seducing and tempting and difficult to curb our passions, but as human beings above the mineral, vegetal and animal kingdom, we have to struggle out of the circle of birth and death. So we must all use our level best and maximum to tread the right path of living divinely and to return to Him, our real Father, God, the Almighty.

N.B. It is a sad that many of the Sufis and other mystics have been opposed by the clerics and only a handful still survive in this material world. When it comes to Hindus as Sanatana Dharma way of living, we find the same treatment by most of the Indians who are going out of the track or against the real way of living. So when you go against the real path of the original living, what will happen is that one is killing and going against his own reality and forgetting his own innerself and against the path of spirituality.

N.B. A special note to all mothers in this world. Many (not all) are responsible for the degradation of human beings. They are not assuming their respected and spiritual responsibility in this world. They are the (Gurus) of the newborn who stay in their wombs for nine months. But when they are pregnant, they never follow the real path with a proper diet; what I mean here is that a balanced food is required in daily life. Now they never follow a discipline of spiritual and art of living. So it is clear that the new-born babe will be out to a subnormal way. Mothers use too much artificial and material objects to bring up and raise their children.

1. The food is not natural to baby and children. Feeding them with artificial food.

2. The way to bring up and raise all in an artificial way.

3. They make their children follow a luxurious life without any discipline.

4. Mould them as the jeweler moulds the gold into all different shapes and jewelleries, Ref: my book, "the children's Yoga."

5. Never use force to guide them. There are spiritual ways to bring up children but mothers themselves never practise or learn them during their conjugal life. Parents miss out all these virtues about bringing up the child in a real and true spiritual path.

6. The Prana (vital force or air). One must learn from PRANA that one should eat to live and not live to eat, that is he should not eat to give strength and nourishment to the senses. The food should be of quality and complete and just sufficient only to feed the flame of life.

7. The soul is all-pervading. It is never affected by the body and the bodily attributes. One should learnt from infinity (that is the blue sky) Akasa which is void and is not affected by clouds, storms, lightning and other objects. So remember that the self-realized soul even lives in the body and should contemplate through his identity with self or soul which is all pervading as well as the blue sky.

8. Too much attachment is bad and should be controlled, as one should control the senses and mind. One should have non-attachment, that is love for anyone. Bear in mind that too much attachment towards anything can cause one's own downfall.

9. A miserable family man is he who has not controlled his senses, who has not withdrawn his senses and mind from worldly objects, who finds delight only in the sexual life and maintains his family in a tense atmosphere. He eventually, comes into conflict with all his relations.

10. The self-realized should always be calm, profound or deep, difficult to fathom, illimitable and immovable or not liable to be perturbed by worldly circumstances like a tranquil ocean.

11. One who has uncontrolled senses, on seeing a woman, the god's Maya (illusion, enchantment created by the Almighty) is being allured by the behaviour and feelings and falls into the blinding darkness and comes to grief, just as the moth falls into the fire. He is a fool who with his mind is allured by wealth, wine, women, gold ornaments, clothes and other things created by illusion (Maya). With such objects of enjoyment, he loses his correct vision and perishes as well like a moth.

12. The miser who hoards wealth, who neither gives nor enjoys his riches, whatever he collects with difficulty is often carried away by some one else.

13. A man gets married to get a woman as partner in life. For the sake of comforts of the body, a person maintains a wife, domestic animals, servants, children, home and relations and amasses wealth with great difficulty. But the body perishes in the end like a tree, creating the seed of a fresh body for him, that he is entangled in the vicious circle of birth and death.

14. He whose senses, mind and intellect do their functions according to the will of God, is freed from the attributes of the body, though dwelling in the body. He is free from the bonds of (Karma) actions though still enveloped by the body.

15. He is a passionate ordinary man who lustfully plays with his follows. Remember that those who find fault with God's creation on earth really have no knowledge of His greatness and glory, as clearly they have never got interested into the practice of Yoga, and as their faults have not been purged by the practice of spirituality such as (Yama and Niyama) and as they have never taken refuge or recourse to the lotus feet of a (Guru), spiritual master; they have no real insight into the Science of Yoga, Adhyatmic Science, genuine living.

16. People who are evil and against the Lord are empty of hope, empty of deeds, empty of wisdom, senseless, are possessed by the devil, are deceitful, brutal, and of demoniac nature. They are enveloped in darkness, take the wrong to be right and see things in a perverted light. These low characters know neither good actions nor renunciations, neither purity nor right conduct, neither truth nor uprightness. They are ignorant and do not know what ought to be done and what ought not to be done. They get deluded by birth after birth, wandering in the worldly mine of material impressions, suffering innumerable illnesses and miseries and they do not attain liberation.

17. A realized character must not get attached to useless mundane objects, although he is placed in the midst of objects with different attributes and though he is placed in the physical body. The mind mainly should remain unaffected by good and evil consequences of the objects. He should be as the air unaffected by the good and bad odour of objects over which it blows.

18. Man should be free from pride, envy, jealousy, without attachment, firmly devoted to the Spiritual Master, free from impatience and intent upon knowing the Truth. He should not find fault with any and should not indulge in unnecessary or idle talk such as gossiping about relatives and wasting precious time with worldly affairs. He should use wisdom to teach his wife, children, kith and kin, and others. He should see all alike because the soul is the same everywhere and through everything the soul shines.

19. An Avatara (incarnation of God) is a descent of God for the ascent of man. He comes with mighty powers to keep up the harmony of the Universe. His works and teachings produce a benign spiritual influence on humans and help them to uplift their divine enfoldment and self-realization. He also comes as a Guru (spiritual Master) to reveal the divinity which is hidden within man and makes him rise above the petty materialistic life of passion and egoism. An Avatar comes on earth only when there is widespread evils within man's characters.

20. There are still some falsehoods of non-believers. The ignorant and thoughtless people always say that the Lord is an ordinary or common man, with human qualities. They even argue that Lord has

come from a lower stage, as they never look or come to know their own innerself and are lost within themselves and become a real slave to the material world. Some their fate. We should not give God anthropomorphic attributes. Love is the essence of life.

The two kinds of Love are:-

1. **Pure Love** – It is like a child who is having breast feeding. Either a girl or a boy has food to survive from the mother's teat or breast. They have only love and there is no sensual pleasure from the mother. This is what we call pure love between children and mother. This is detachment of mind.
2. **Pleasure or sensual love**. This is the attachment and have the same thing for enjoying sensual pleasure. It is like a man and a woman having sexual and lustful pleasure by using the breast of a woman to caress it or suck or kiss it. This is done only for pleasure and sensual gratification.

The two characteristics of Sacrifice are:
This also is a sort of detachment.
1. One sort of Sacrifice is to do it only for God and just help others disinterestedly. It is only a one-way traffic. This characteristic is really very near to divinity.
2. This second sort of Sacrifice is done either to expect something at any moment, either soon or in the future. It is growing a seed to expect fruit from it. If we do an action now to expect an advantage

in the future, this is a two-way traffic. This one has attachment and selfishness.

Man needs a balanced diet, which means that the food should have all the minerals, vitamins, carbohydrate, fat, protein, starching equivalent proportion in the daily food. It does not mean that one must have meat, fish and eggs in this diet to get the good balanced diet. On the contrary, if one can refrain from non-vegetarian food, the better for one's own health.

My advice is to the old people after mainly 60 years old.
Children should be taught that they are not the body and mind complex only, they are the spirit as well.

Nowadays, many intellectual people have read and learnt sacred scriptures and they just lecture on them like parrots, but really there are few who put them into daily and regular practice. This is one of the reasons for the spread of evil in our modern civilization.

The most incredible thing is that people over 60, instead of going deeply in spiritual life to know their own innerself, are indulging in materialism, apart from a few.

"They never come out of this circle of birth and death, they are taking birth and get retrograted into the lower species and they are dying with all sorts of mental degradation effects and lower life."

He who is full of knowledge of wisdom is eternally free; he is the one who does not expect any reward for his good actions. He knows himself as well as others. He who expects the fruits of his actions is ignorant and always bound.

The wise one is not conditioned by the body, though is in the body, like a man aroused from dream.

The ordinary man who has a wrong notion is conditioned by the body like one in the dreaming state. So the ignorant man identifies himself with the body like the man in dream.

The foolish man who allows his sense of taste to override him, who is stupefied with the charms of taste and delicacies by the turbulent and greedy tongue, meets with horrible death. The tongue or the love of taste is the most difficult to conquer. If the sense of taste is controlled, all the other senses are controlled. One cannot become master of his organs until he controls the organ of taste. No man can be said to have conquered his senses unless his organ of taste is totally curbed. Thoughtful men subdue their senses by fasting.

For the sake of the comfort of the body, a person maintains a wife, domestic animals, servants, children, home and relations and amasses wealth with great difficulty and is often a miser and mean. This body perishes in the end like a tree, creating the seed of a fresh body for him.

Taste is the worst enemy of man. The tongue drags him to one side and the thirst to another, the organs of reproduction to some other, the skin, the stomach and ear in some other direction; the sense of smell in one direction, the fickle eye to something else, the tendency for work draws him to something else and every other physical organ in a different direction of activity. The senses sap his very life blood, even as the many wives of one husband the "King Dasaruth with his tree wives."

A person who is stabilized in soul consciousness and God consciousness, considers all worldly things and objects of pleasure like garbage...For him there is no difference between gold and stone.

Spiritually, the death of the ego is the emergence of Divinity:- That which divides you from the Lord Almighty is the worst enemy (Ego). This ego is like a veil between one and God. But the sooner this Ego disintegrates, the quicker one comes face to face with the Almighty (God). So one is in a complete detachment from illusionary world and of the "I" and "Mine" These two words of "I" and "Mine" bind the individual soul.

The true path to Yoga and spirituality is the coin with positive terms which liberates a man by practising of "Not I, Not mine" and finally he attains the highest goal of freedom and liberation or self-realization in this only human form.

To have satisfaction, Love and acceptance of one's life, such a one is really a spiritual man.

In my book the children's Yoga, "SALUTATION TO SUN", one will learn more about the upraising or bringing up of children in a spiritual method. But as already pointed out, parents are moulding their offspring by transforming them into complete material beings. The little child of God is dramatically changed from an innocent attitude to an unrealistic approach of life. It is not bad to make them intelligent and intellectual scientifically and materially, but what is more important is to educate the child about his spirituality. Children should be taught: where they come from? What have they come to do? Where are they going? Actually, we are just making the young like electric robots.

What is worst is to see the parents giving the bad example by watching T.V programmes most of the time with all sorts of rubbish, at times erotic films. All these indecent postures do not contribute to the uplift of people.

Finally, parents greatly encourage children to consume very bad and wrong foods, mainly in the morning and during the days. This is causing bad health to children and the mental attitude of the children becomes bound with material living. The children have no serenity of mind from their childhood. Bad habits of foods make the children may be so- called intelligent but with a fragmented and restless mind through life.

We are fashioning a complete material world from the cradle to the grave. We forget that man has the intellect and the spirit, while animals have instincts. Only the mind makes man either a human or a demon. Man should make proper use of his mind and body so that he can protect his health. If you want an healthy body and mind you should cultivate knowledge of wisdom and the control of the senses. The pure mind must be supreme in all works and actions in whatever situation. Therefore, it is extremely important to keep the mind healthy and pure with pure and good thoughts. If the mind is not healthy, then the body also becomes unhealthy. However 99.999% people do not pay attention to this fact, and neglect the spiritual in an over-secularised and material world. After all, it is mind that places man above all other creatures. (No mind, no man). Our mind, can be the best friend or our worst enemy. Control its fluctuations, calm down its evil-prosperity, neither suppress nor flatter it. Just be a witness to its doings. "This world exists due to mind. No mind, no world."

CHAPTER 11
CONCLUSION

This is to conclude that yoga as a science is the only therapeutic process of self-treatment and it also helps to cure the illnesses and diseases from their roots. In my opinion, the world can get away from these catastrophic and calamitous situation through the yogic concepts by performing proper yoga practice, like Asanas and Pranayama, Rhythmic breathing, Suryanamaskar, relaxation, concentration, proper diet, and finally a clear knowledge in the life of an individual.

However, to have a better world in the future, it is up to the individual to proceed with the yogic therapy in his daily life. The main importance of the Yogic concepts can be practised better if the individual agrees with the point that the mind is the only organ that activates, governs and controls the whole body. In fact, one needs an excellent body and mind to carry on with yoga conception, but one more important thing is of great use to an individual, this is the harmonization of these two faculties. To achieve this harmony, body and mind, the individual must develop and acquire proper knowledge about the concepts, theories and the philosophies of life. By practising the Yogic ideas in daily life, an individual becomes a maker of his own destiny and life. One need no longer the mercy of others, worldly and heavenly. It is only the practical method that can bestow the complete above benefits to an individual.

From the Yoga point of view, an individual is his own master, that is a very powerful being. He is a dependent of his ownself. What one wants to do or be, one will do or be. One is responsible for what one is today and the future; no power in this world can stop one from fulfilment because one already pocesses all the power, energy, life force and will-power within oneself.

You have already been misled and misguided by others blindly to believe and rely on the superiority of external power. However, Yoga stops you here and makes you think in a new way. Don't let yourself be misguided again any more, as great harm has already been caused on relying on external factors. Furthermore, don't waste any time. Stand on your own feet. Open your mind and find out the Truth for yourself. Believe in nothing until you find it out for yourself and believe that inner strength (Satyagraha) only is life. Yoga follows a logic, what an individual has done can always be done by another individual. One is as good as anyone born in the past or now. But the only difference between characters is because of the difference in actions, knowledge, efforts and know-how. If an individual follows others, just do the same or copy as others, the result will be definitely the same.

Unfortunately, many individuals blame themselves and become capable of the ideas of sin, fate, guilt and evil. The individuals are misled and torture themselves ignorantly. An individual should always be positive in whatever situation he is, never get trapped by the vicious character of negative thoughts. From yoga point of view, KARMA YOGA plays the most important phase in an individual in day to day life. So yoga disposes the notions of inaction and dependence. No individual should refrain from actions.

But to act even an evil action is better than no action at all. Yoga teaches one not to runaway form work and worldly life, no matter the hard works or difficult problems or the opinions of others. One should, indeed, differentiate and distinguish from the desirable and undesirable.

One should have a very good knowledge of discrimination. Don't forget that evil and good are the sides of the same coin; if an individual does good actions, he will reap the good fruits and if he does bad or evil actions, he will reap the same rotten fruits during his human life or he will be born and has a degraded life.

Evidently enough, we all commit mistakes, but one must learn from them and correct them so that in the future we don't repeat these mistakes. That's why the words "Forgive" and "Forget" and "Tolerance" must be put into practice, inorder that one can discriminate and become good individuals.

Sin and evils are but only mistakes and errors done by a weak individual. Bear in mind that all errors and mistakes can be corrected in one's life. So we have no right to condemn! KRISHNA says:- If one can correct and discriminate his mistakes and errors, he is elevated to the grade of a saint.

Furthermore human should tolerate and encourage such character and precise him and let him ascend in society and during his whole life itself.

If one finds there is an error in one's doing, correct it and be reformed. That really is a spiritual victory in one's life.

Finally, yoga is a science to make man better, mentally and physically. If the practice is carried sincerely and with love, then the fruits will be definitely sweet. Yoga can be put into practice by anyone, man, woman, child and youngster and regardless of races or colours, creed or community. It is meant for everyone in this universe.

Thus this text covers a range of simple yoga techniques which are meant for common or ordinary people. These techniques can easily be practised by any one in one's daily life and might help him to face diseases and stress and depression of the daily life in this hectic and competitive modern life.

I bless you who practise them with certitude for a happy living.

Religion is to live with fear of God but Spirituality is to live with Love of God. And the revelation of God can be done within everyone. "You ARE GOD AND HE IS IN YOU, REVEAL HIM."

PEACE TO THE WORLD
1. LOKA SAMASTA SUKHINO BHAVANTU

May all the worlds be happy. May all the beings be happy. May non suffer from grief. PRAYER FOR LIGHT AND SUN.

2. ASATO MAA SATGAMAYA

TAMASO MAA JYOTIRGAMAYA

MRITYOR MAA AMRITAM GAMAYA

Lead me from untruth to TRUTH

Lead me from Darkness to light

Lead me from death to immortality

AUM SHANTIH, SHANTIH, SHANTIH

PEACE, PEACE, PEACE.

However, the true happiness is not in the objects, but in the state or behaviour of the mind which is free and independent of these material objects. The bliss or real happiness is an inherent quality of our Inner-Self and can be free, if we learn to turn our attention from the external world, that is materialism to the inner world that is our true self and follow the yoga paths, such as Karma, Bhakti, Hatha, Meditation and so on. Nowadays, in this material world, people think that without objects to strive after, people would be in a situation of emptiness, boredom, meaninglessness or dullness. This misunderstanding is found upon viewing objects as the main things of satisfaction in this world. People do not have the realization that joy and true happiness can be searched or experienced without material objects. The origin of joy, happiness and peace or bliss is within all of us and we do not have to run after anyone or anywhere outside to get it. So stay wherever you are, just one must have the

215

determination within and practise spirituality on a daily regular basis, that is all one needs to do, but with sincerity and love within as well.

Remember as well that we should not have to abandon the world or hate material objects. One should practise detachment of mind and control of the monkey mind, discrimination, discipline of diet, some breathing exercises, few postures in one's daily life. Really nothing is impossible, study the life of Jesus, Muhammad, Ram, Krishna etc.. They never led a retired life or lived as a hermit. They all lived in this material world, but with disciplines as I did mention above.

Material objects themselves are not the problem, it is the attachment to them which brings all these problems to human life. So by practising Yoga, one maintains a healthy attitude towards material objects. Actually, one is encouraged to enjoy the experience and to use material objects to reach one's goals, but we should abstain from becoming attached to them. One should utilize them (objects) as one's servants and not allow them to become one's masters and let one be dominated by them. One should use them at his minimum in one's daily life.

Remember if one develops detachment and dispassion or discrimination in a yoga way of life towards worldly objects and events, then pleasure and pain automatically lose their hold on him. He is relieved of the rein of pleasure and pain. Then one develops a complete attitude of equanimity towards all pleasures and pains; furthermore he remains equipoise in all the opposite situations, is neither excited by gains, nor stressed by losses. If the practice of spiritualism is done sincerely and properly, no world situation will disturb the inner peace and balance.

Gita says: "For the pleasures that come from the world, bear in them sorrows to come. They come and go, they are transient not in them, do the wise rejoice."

Really to say, the wise man never craves for sensual pleasures deliberately and thus stays free from the sorrows and pains associated with them, because pain exists only when there is pleasure. There is a simple practice and formula to carry on daily, that is if one doesn't want pains, avoid running after useless pleasures also.

Therefore rather than becoming attached to the sensations of pleasures while rejecting pains, simply look upon them both like a detached observer and take note of their coming and passing with full control of the monkey mind. Callous people are ignorant, hypocrites, selfish, and are completely slaves to materialism. They are also full of likes and dislikes with a vacillating mind, and they create enemies around themselves. Instead they should practise neutrality and be indifferent to circumstance so as to come out of the dark veil of this modern material life.

Learn to live within the innerself joy with a peaceful mind rather than in the excitements derived from sense gratifications and satisfactions. What we all face in this present life is ordered by our past and how we face them alone determines the future progress and growth of our inner personality.

One has to face the world as it is, and act as to be at peace within the Inner-Self and to be in a joyous sense of inner contentment and satisfaction.

Bear in mind that there is nothing in this world which happens by chance, luck or accident. There is always a reason for everything which occurs to anyone. One is bound by a great relationship of the law of cause and effect. For every effect, there is a cause and for every cause there is an effect; this is the inscrutable law of all that is.

Actually a sincere disciple should not involve his attention and interest to be squandered into the channels of worldly affairs, pleasures and passions. Nowadays trivial pleasures and idle talks are mainly based on the five issues:-

1. Wine, women, wealth, enemies and pleasures. In any gathering or function, people discuss only these exclusive topics. So people get detracted and derailed on their journey from spiritual path by these wasteful talks on these above mentioned issues. Avoid such harmful talks. And let all our talks be on the spiritual topics, i.e the nature of Truth, the sorrows of this world of plurality, the lot of the ego, the ways of freedom, the realization of self-control, the marvellous life divine and the glories of self-realization and Science of Yoga, mainly for the body and mind complex.

Be impartial, neutral or indifferent wisely, whatever one may call it. The spiritual path needs not only meditation and good actions, but also the necessity of the balanced psychological health. To achieve and fulfil a spiritual life, one must be careful about the negative qualities, that are the veils and can destroy the peace and happiness and relationships with others and keep one away from the Almighty.

Spiritual life is really difficult, but not impossible. Without sincerity and wholeheartedness along the straight and narrow path, it is very difficult to seek for Him, the Lord. One cannot attain Him, without maximum sacrifice and mainly by erasing the body and mind "Ego" and this ego which again stands as a black wall between the disciple and God. (Guru)

The I-ness is the self-prison, so the fake pride derived from attaching complete importance and forgetting that the Almight is the only doer. The time one indulges in pride, one is trading to his downfall in spirituality.

Remember many people are world famous, wealthy, intelligent, celebrities, stars with name and fame but many still end their lives miserably as drug-addicts, neurotics and some even commit suicide, and die with the terrible fate of birth and death, that is they are coming back, retrograding into animalism. All this because they do not pay attention to their Inner-Self.

Now one should not be dishonest to himself and to God. Dishonesty is a big mistake and a sin in one's daily life. One cannot be dishonest and have his mind with God. It will be impossible to have one's feet in two different boats, that is one leading towards the truth and the next in the opposite direction.

Now be careful that discrimination must be a guide in this world of relativity. And try to surrender oneself to Him. Repent sincerely to God. "Oh Lord Almighty, I was impatient, I lost my temper I know it is wrong, because I am no longer at peace within my heart. Forgive me."

Don't play tricks with God by using a two-face, one in truth and the latter in untruth; you are just fooling your ownself ignorantly. One must have patience and loving determination to win God in one's daily life. This is an ordinary behaviour of human reaction in this hectic attitude of life. People are all guilty of turning impatient at any time, mainly when they are under pressure, tension and fear, characteristics of our fretful modern pace of living.

Hatred and resentment are two cousins. Hatred and resentment destroy one's spiritual life. The moment you allow yourself to become influenced by these two, you lose your complete awareness of Him, the Almighty. Eradicate them from one's consciousness and try one's level best to throw them out if they want to grasp you.

Jealousy and envy are of the same coin. It is clear that when we are one with God, we don't find any cause for jealousy and envy. An individual is happy with what he has, he recognizes that it comes from Him the Almighty. Jealousy and envy are very common nowadays with worldly minded people.

It is said that you should keep eyes on your own thing and never be concerned with what anyone else is doing. To seek God, one has to be very alert, mentally and physically. We sow what we reap. Laziness is the worst negative quality that one must overcome. If one wants to succeed in searching for God, one can be forgiven for his physical laziness, but not for his mental spiritual side. For mental laziness means a lack of will-power or enthusiasm for spirituality.

If one does not perform one's work, meditation, Yoga and other responsibilities with a wholehearted enthusiasm, with a divine motivation, one will never reach God, nor the true happiness one is searching for; it is impossible. However, no one can give him that spirit. It has to come from within. And one has to change one's mental behaviour.

Now we have procrastination, which is a tough by-product of laziness. A procrastinate person always says no today I will do it tomorrow, but today let me be what I am. And this can carry on all the days of one's life. Therefore, one who keeps postponing things never achieves his goal. One must do the very best now, today and everyday. Negative and positive thinking are the two sides of the same coin. One side of the coin, for example, can not exist without the other. Similarly, there are two ways to look at every situation, positively and negatively. Always be very certain to look in the positive side. Never allow oneself to wallow in negative actions, for if someone does so, he will have no inner peace, and will find it very hard indeed to be with Him, God. It is clear that the mind of negative people are always restless and unease.

221

Remember that positive thinking makes the difference between the ordinary man and the divine man. And never allow the mind to be dragged down by outer circumstances of this illusionary world.

The negative and vulgar thoughts come clearly from the sub-conscious mind. The mind is divided into three parts:
1. consciousness/unconsciousness
2. Sub-consciousness, and
3. Super-consciousness which are clearly explained in my book of "Mind/thoughts/ Ayurvedic and diseases."

The subconsciousness is a part of mind which is like a store-keep all the good and bad things from past life till now. So one must know and try hard to make it clean. It is a repository of all the past experiences including negative thoughts, gossip, worldliness, affairs of the past and thus the beginning of one's life.

When one tries to meditate, mainly the beginners, they get difficulties because that sub-consciousness is like a glass of dark muddy water but with yoga, gradually the dark thoughts begin to settle or vanish and the clear water of divine perception starts appearing.

The conscious mind is natural, but with negative thinking, thoughts, gossip, jealousy, envy, hatred, worries and all negative qualities, its purity is obscured. So when one learns to tranquil and subdue the mind with

Yoga, meditation, one will find that the natural consciousness and sub-consciousness again become purified.

Remember as well if the mind is filled with negative and busy catering to any of these other psychological liabilities such as worldly affairs etc.. one will not be able to have relationship with God and love for God. Although God is within everything, but first the innerself should realize Him, then will it be possible to see Him everywhere and in everything.

We all come from Him and we are all his "image", so one must repeat this to Lord over and over again in one's daily life:-

"I have come into this world to change myself. Help me Oh Lord, give me whatever discipline, will-power, faith you know I need. All I know is that I love you. I want you, I want to perfect myself so that I can find you within my "Innerself."

Try to call Him lovingly, even if at times the body and mind and ego try to drag one down, do not be dismayed. Carry on calling Him silently, give me love for thee, Reveal Thyself, Reveal Thyself.

Finally, never stop to keep on trying to do better to spiritualize your life in every way you can. The only difference between a saint and an ordinary common man is that the saint never gives up trying even when the goal is attained.

One must be detached, measured or neutral in the daily life. To have a peaceful mind, one must learn to be detached, with the mind being discriminate and wise, but not to be indifferent ignorantly.

Common and ordinary people are the real slaves of this material world and they never get satisfied and practise the purity of love daily. They are always thinking that they must enjoy and have pleasures and use the maximum material enjoyments at any opportunity that comes before them.

Nowadays, work has become money-wise, and the works are not being done as duties. With this way of life, people are becoming mere slaves of this money-wise world. Eventually they become fragmented and their mind is attached till their death and would never come out from the circle of birth and death. Their mind is being tortured by success and failure, bad and good, happiness and sorrow, which are the two sides of a coin. They are running after all this false world and due to this false attitude, they completely forget themselves, I mean their innerself.

Materially, people have changed their concept of religion in this modern era. They use it for their own gain and they have changed this Pure Love which is the main core of religion into an egocentric character and now most are not spiritually minded. Religion without love is deplorable as this is nowadays. Most claries of the institutionalized, religions are for money and often mere fanatics.

Actually if you are a scientist or an intellectual, this makes you become a worldly man, but spirituality makes a man become Godman or ManGod in this world. But it is pity to see only a handful of real spiritual men in this world.

It is due to ignorance and misguidedness by the parents and foreparents, who have followed the rites, rituals and dogmas and most of the people fall in the same trap of meaningless ritualism only and the coming generation will be a complete misfit to Religion and the Spiritual.

What I mean is that the blind are leading the blind in this illusionary world. And there is only outside evolution and there is not spiritual involution in human characters.

With such trends, this world is full of egoistics, hypocrites and selfish characters. This is occurring because people are too much attached to material objects.

Worldly people are very worried and their nervous systems and mind are shattered and sickened. Although they live (exist) for 100 hundred years, what difference it makes, nothing, because they are empty bags of shattered nerves. This world is a stage from where they should practise and lead a spiritual life to go back to the Divinity from where they come, but instead they get themselves bound in the circle of birth and death.

There are many who think they are very intelligent because they know all about this illusionary world with their pleasures and indulgences. They eat everything without discipline and many drink alcohol every night and their concern is too much with worldly pleasures, family and they never get time to realize their inner-self. They are living but how?(only existing). This they have to ask themselves. To Mingle with this sort of people becomes difficult to realize yourself, but in spirituality one must detach and discriminate the main thing "the mind."

The mind is the heaven or the hell. It is up to you to choose which one you should choose, but it is very sad to see how many people follow the wrong path! Most of them choose the complete wrong side of "I and Mine" path which leads to the downfall of humans

.

As one is involved with the strong attachment to husband, wife, children, relations, friends, wealth, women and wine in this material world, one will have to suffer and will never be at peace within. It is because the two words of "I" and "Mine" will devour his mental attitude and behaviour. Finally it becomes difficult to detach the mind, so he gets entangled in the net of birth and death. He will never be free and get liberated.

He has to live with the vicissitudes of life. He is caught in the vice-like grip of the two words of "I" and "Mine" business and this will be his fate, but he should try to start landing on the path of this Science of Yoga. This should be his daily part and parcel of his human life.

But once one gets involved in this business of worldly and material habits, it becomes attached and entangled and one can't come out, because the attachment to this illusion (MAYA) world is so strong that people find it difficult to come out of it. But there is a way which could be practised. I know it is very hard but it is possible, only if people start to introduce this Science of Yoga in every walk of life. Unfortunately, the power (MAYA) is so attractive and powerful that in the end, they let themselves become the slaves of this illusionary and material world which is in a constant flux. It is due to that wrong situation that nature is degrading to a worse state.

But there is always a way to get out, if everyone tries to discover his own reality and truth through this practice of Yoga, and try to go and seek for the Innerself. This is the Reality and Truth, then we can reach liberation and free ourselves from the unreality of this material world.

Unfortunately, people are greatly influenced and attracted by the force of material lures and in the end, they fall in this circle of birth and death which is a road without end. In reality, there is a spiritual way to get out of the opposites and the twin terms that bring to liberation. The twin terms are "NOT I, NOT MINE" this brings freedom and liberation (Moksa).

By renouncing those twin terms, one can get ultimate peace, joy, bliss and believe me all problems come to their ends. Finally, the grieves of the soul of the spirit and of the individual are definitely eliminated.

"As long as you are there (i.e the ego is there), God can't be. Only when you are not there, "I mean the Ego," God is. Both can't live together. So to attain God, one has to lose oneself (i.e. the Ego). Why people don't attain God, it is crystal clear that they don't want to lose themselves and merge to become (NOBODY). The reality is that the feeling of (NOBODY) naturally makes one EVERYBODY, without any effort on his part.

This turning to (NOBODY) or loss of the 'Ego' is not a state of emptiness or boredom as most people misunderstand it. It is rather a state of the explainable or indescribable bliss, joy and peace within oneself. It is when one attains this awareness of purity as advocated by the great sages that one is happy with God. Shankaracharya, the great sage of that time, declared. "Aham Brahmasmi", i.e "I am God." This is the awareness of the Divine which springs in complete loss of Ego when the pure "I" shines in someone.

So here I advise any one to practise Yoga, inorder just to know this purity of "I" or pure consciousness. As one goes deeper in it, one can become transformed. And it is the highest state of awareness which removes all the suffering and delusion of being. It can also be called the true and original nature or the innermost consciousness. People's Ego or the false "I" is simply a super imposition over the original nature and is not a permanent part of people, and can be disposed of as soon as people wake up from their sleep of ignorance, hypocrisy, selfishness, Egohood and all kinds of material concerns of this modern era.